GARLIC FOR HEALTH

DAVID ROSER

THE GARLIC RESEARCH BUREAU

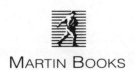

MARTIN BOOKS

Published by Martin Books
Simon & Schuster International Group
Fitzwilliam House
32 Trumpington Street
Cambridge CB2 1QY

ISBN 0 85941 674 7

First published 1990

Text © 1990 David Roser
Illustrations © 1990 Woodhead-Faulkner (Publishers) Ltd
Design: Merchant Design
Illustration: Ken Brasier
Typesetting: Goodfellow & Egan, Cambridge
Printed and bound by: BPCC Wheatons Ltd, Exeter

Contents

Foreword   5

1 Garlic - a medicine
   for more than five
   thousand years   6

2 Garlic for a long and
   healthy life   22

3 How garlic works - an
   easy garlic chemistry
   lesson   33

4 Time for action -
   getting garlic
   goodness into your life   51

5 Garlic for today and
   tomorrow   77

   Appendix A: A window on current garlic
   research   89
   Appendix B: Useful addresses and
   references   94
   Index   95

Foreword

Garlic is unique in its potential for aiding human health. There is no other plant whose activities are so wide-ranging across such a host of different health areas. In the past this Jack-of-all-trades reputation has been damaging to garlic's image, because without a full and understandable explanation of garlic's multi-faceted chemical make-up, it was hard to believe in its apparent ability to tackle a wide range of health problems.

Additionally, it used to be thought that cooked garlic was less potent than raw garlic in its effectiveness, and that preparations of garlic, such as oils and powders, were not as effective as the whole raw plant. We now know that this is not the case.

It is important that garlic's credibility is restored, not on the basis of anecdotes and stories of miracle cures, but by invoking relevant scientific work carried out by professionally qualified researchers.

I have been involved in detail with garlic in all its forms for nearly ten years and can contrast attitudes towards it in the late seventies and now. An enormous change has taken place, and garlic is now regarded with a great deal more seriousness.

This book is intended to be a practical guide to the use of garlic in a wide range of different situations; garlic for your health and in your cookery, for your pets and in your garden.

I need no convincing of just how important garlic is to very many people, who've seen in their own lives the changes (some quite dramatic) that garlic has made to their health. We now buy and use more garlic per head of population than ever before in Britain, and this trend is set to accelerate yet again over the next few years.

The growth of garlic-based preparations has been quite breath-taking too, with around 1 million people regularly using garlic preparations during 1989 in the United Kingdom.

Garlic goes on proving itself every day, both scientifically and in our daily lives. I hope my book will help to expand its use yet further.

David Roser
The Garlic Research Bureau

1

Garlic – a medicine for more than 5,000 years

We know for a fact, from a combination of written records and artefacts left in tombs, that garlic in one form or another has been an important medicine in most of the world's great civilisations. Of course, the use of garlic must have been widespread for many thousands of years before the first surviving records, which refer to garlic as a well established remedy for a number of ailments. Perhaps the most interesting findings are that the uses to which garlic was put appear to have been very similar amongst populations who had no known contacts with one another, and who therefore must have discovered garlic's benefits through trial and, no doubt, error, on their own.

THE GARLIC FAMILY

Many different kinds of garlic can be traced in these historical records. The genus *Allium* (the family name for garlic and onions) comprises some 600 different species and is found virtually everywhere throughout the world.

Also belonging to this family are chives, leeks, potatoes, shallots and common onions. Amongst the true garlics there are many interesting variations, such as rocambole. This is also called 'serpent garlic', due to its coiled stems, or 'giant garlic'. It can be used in place of culinary garlic, although it is seldom grown these days. Rocambole is believed to have originated from Denmark. Other types are 'crow garlic', 'field garlic' and 'great-headed garlic'. All these grow wild and are self-perpetuating.

In European countries, wild garlic has always grown, especially in marshland fringes and wetlands. Its old countryside names include 'sauce alone' and 'hedge garlic'. 'Jack-by-the-hedge' is a relative of the mustard plant that has a strong garlicky flavour, and was a favourite flavouring in soups and stews in the Middle Ages.

Perhaps the best known of the uncultivated garlics is 'ransom' or 'ram's garlic' – so called because of its heavy, lingering pungency. It is very prolific, especially in England, and can be seen in damp woodlands where it scents the air

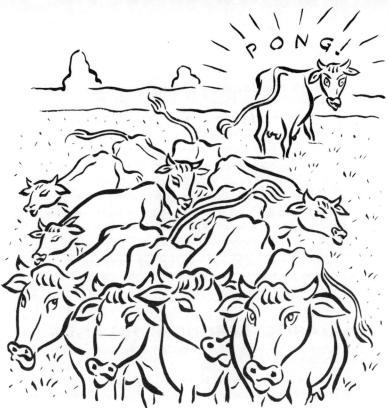

Cows that eat garlic are easily spotted!

for some considerable distance. Its name suggests a very unfavourable comparison with the smell of the wild ram, which, like the billy goat, can be an animal to be avoided unless you're wearing a gas mask! Indeed, farmers and stockmen are very careful to ensure that grazing cattle are kept well away from both ransom and wild garlic because their high sulphur content will taint the milk of cattle and flavour the meat; this takes several days or even weeks to decline naturally. Ransom and wild garlic were undoubtedly the basis of garlic medicines and flavourings prior to the introduction of true culinary garlic.

ORIGINS OF THE NAME

So where did the name 'garlic' originate? 'Gar' is believed to have meant 'spear' or lance in Old English and 'lic' is a leek. Garlic's proper name is *Allium sativum*; *Allium* is believed to derive from the Celtic *all* which simply means 'smelly', whilst *sativum* just means 'grown' or cultivated.

Other old names for garlic abound. Garlic was believed to

be a cure for bites from mammals such as shrews and mice, as well as for stings from scorpions and even for snake bites. It was believed both to counteract the effects of poisons and to help remove them from the body. The Latin word for such actions was *thieracus* or antidote. This, it is thought, may have been corrupted in common use and became 'treacle'. Garlic was thus known as 'Poor man's treacle'! But it had other names too, some of which are redolent of magic and mystery. 'The Devil's Posy', 'Poor Man's Camphor', 'Witches' Poison', 'The Fruit of Love' and probably the best known 'The Stinking Rose'. All of these names have their roots in thousands of years of myth and legend that have grown up around and accompanied garlic wherever it has been used.

GARLIC THROUGH THE AGES

The history of garlic is full of wonder and mystery and more has been written about this little plant than virtually any other single herb. It weaves its way through magic, myth and fable and has been involved in religion, politics and power, not to mention the odd miracle here and there.

So garlic has had the attention of the great and good for thousands of years. As we get ready to enter the twenty-first century, new scientific validations of many of the traditionally believed virtues of 'garlicke' are being made in laboratories and hospitals throughout the world. There's more about this in chapter 2, but first let us look at the enormous and very entertaining history of this miracle plant. This is an epic adventure story with all of the elements of a first-class thriller: magic, intrigues, discoveries, miraculous cures, facts, fables and fallacies and most of all, garlic's shining presence through countless ages, helping, healing and supporting millions of long-gone peoples in their fight against diseases and infections.

GARLIC IN CHINA: ORIGINS AND FIRST USES

Whilst garlic and onions have been cultivated in the Middle East and Asia for thousands of years, it is to China that we turn first to examine the earliest uses of garlic. The garlic that you buy now in your supermarket or greengrocer probably originated from China. This 'culinary' garlic is likely to have first evolved in the mysterious and little known wildernesses of the landlocked northern and western parts of that gigantic land, somewhere in the foothills of the vast mountain ranges such as the Pamirs and Tsien Shan (Heavenly Mountains). These peaks guard the entrances to China from the rest of Asia, with only precipitous passes allowing access to Afghanistan and points west. Every year, their melting snows cascade as the purest waters into the foothills bordering the great plains which roll on to the Lop Nor desert. Where those waters finally drain away, they deposit fine alluvial rock grains, rich in minerals and nutrients, which over centuries and with cultivation and irrigation have become fertile and abundant oases.

Garlic is believed 'always' to have grown here. The cultivation of garlic is thought to have spread from here to Southern Russia. It is also believed that garlic 'escaped' from here some time around 3000 BC, in the direction of India. From around 700 BC the Chinese began to supply silks to the growing and wealthy populace of Greece and probably the camel and yak trains also carried garlic and other spices such as ginger. The oases in north-west China where garlic was cultivated became part of the Great Silk Road, the major trading route from China to Europe.

This trade with the Greeks carried on for at least another five hundred years. The Romans subsequently also took silks, porcelains and spices from the Chinese, and they may have taken garlic too, but it is also possible that they imported garlic from Egypt.

Garlic had great cultural importance in China itself, and was highly prized. Evidence for its importance can be found in linguistics: the Chinese word for garlic, 'suan', is written as a single sign, which often indicates that the object was commonplace early on in the evolution of the language. Together with ginger, garlic was a key constituent of oriental cuisines, particularly in China. A fifth-century AD treatise on agriculture describes the cultivation for cooking of garlic, onions, shallots and spring onions, and says that garlic was the most important of these. Garlic also features in traditional Chinese medicine, used in combination with a vast and complex arsenal of 'healing' plants.

So what did the ancient Chinese use garlic for? Longevity seems to have been one major benefit that they believed in.

An ancient sage is quoted as follows

> 'When you are 50 years old then you should eat
> garlic for 50 days and you will live for a further
> 50 years.'

Garlic was considered a 'heating' herb, and was thus used
against tumours and for diseases and conditions which were
considered to be 'cold': problems such as clammy hands and
damp skin; mucal secretions; tuberculosis; rheumatism and
coughs and colds. It was probably also used for animals as a
vermifuge or wormer, and to guard against parasites both
internal and external, such as ringworm and lice in humans.
The Chinese very seriously believed that garlic had a part to
play in most human diseases, both as a curative and as a
preventive. Clay models of garlic have been excavated with
the so-called 'terracotta army', so garlic was obviously
revered as part of a warrior's diet. Now modern science is
able to review these old ways, and today new and important
trial results are coming out of China showing that garlic can
indeed perform miracles in diseases such as tumours, heart
disease and problem infections. More of this later.

SOUTHERN ASIA:
GARLIC SPREADS ITS INFLUENCE

To get to the advanced civilisations of the Mediterranean
basin – such as Egypt and Greece – where abundant
evidence for garlic's central role in health begins to pile up,
knowledge of garlic's cultivation and use had to spread from
India and China across the wild lands of modern
Afghanistan and southern Russia, and through present-day
Iran, Iraq and Syria. Not much is known about garlic's
history in these lands, but it was valued for its health-giving
and food-enhancing properties by the various peoples of the
area. The Sumerians and Babylonians (c. 4000 BC) used
garlic against such terrible diseases as leprosy, and against
the regular epidemics of such killers as cholera and typhoid.
There are also references to the healing properties of garlic
in the Talmud, the ancient holy writings of the Israelites.

If we now turn to look at Ancient Egypt, we can find a
fully documented history of the use made of garlic by
ancient civilisations.

Ancient Egypt:
The first documentary evidence

A variety of culinary garlic is native to the rich alluvial soils of the Nile delta. Garlic has always had a reputation for giving stamina and strength to its users and there is a delightful story that is told in connection with the building of the Great Pyramid of Cheops at Gizeh. The workers (and not all of them were slaves) were given relatively good food, and garlic, onions and radishes were part of their rations. For some reason, the supplies of garlic ran out and the reaction of the work force was instant: they withdrew their labour. No garlic – then no work! They knew well that garlic and onions gave them strength and stamina and protected them from illnesses and fevers. Perhaps they also knew that regular intakes of garlic kept away biting insects such as gnats and mosquitos and thus (unbeknown to them) prevented malaria and other fevers which must have been rife.

It would have been well understood that those who regularly took particular foods in their diet were in some way given protection, although the reasons were unknown. This understanding is, of course, the whole basis of ancient and traditional medicine – a sort of centuries-old clinical trial of what did and what didn't work.

The Greeks called the Egyptians 'the bread eaters'. In the productive lands of the Nile Valley, flooded each year with a fresh layer of fertile soil, they grew grain in enormous quantities. During the milling of this into coarse flours for baking, the sandstone millwheels would progressively break down, adding fine silica grains to the flour. A regular consumption of these did little to help dental health and the average Egyptian had real problems with badly worn-down teeth. This in turn led to abscessing and the only remedy for such painful infections was garlic. Garlic also could be used – crushed to a paste – over the offending tooth to alleviate the pain, and must have saved the sanity of many an agonised Egyptian in past times. A recent study carried out into the dentition of mummified Egyptians has confirmed severe abscessing and sinal bone erosion – a really painful and potentially life-threatening condition if not treated early.

It was also the habit of the Egyptians to bury their dead with a supply of food, clothing and other essentials of life to ensure that the after life could be led in the same style as

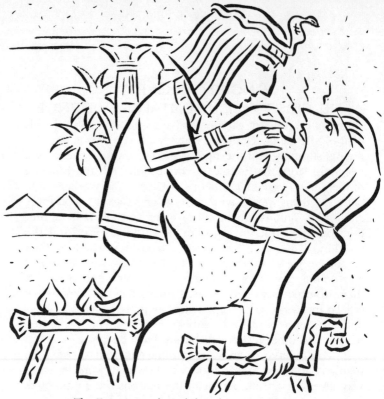

The Egyptians relieved dental agony with garlic.

before death. Realistic clay models of whole garlic bulbs have been found in Egyptian tombs from as long ago as 5000 BC, along with models of wheat, olives and dates. Garlic was obviously a dietary staple like these better-known foods. In the tomb of Tutankhamen – a relatively insignificant boy-king born at the highest point of the power and influence of Egypt and buried in 1500 BC – several complete cloves of real garlic were found.

In the famous Ebers papyrus, which also dates from around 1500 BC, mention is made of garlic's importance in remedies for heart problems, tumours and bites of animals and insects. Some 30 recipes for medicines are given which contain this powerful herb.

THE MEDITERRANEAN AREA

From Egypt, a well-developed trade existed with the kingdom of the Minoans, who developed a civilisation in Crete of considerable power. For some 700 years from 3000 BC the Minoans ruled in the Mediterranean and undoubtedly carried garlic from Egypt into Palestine and throughout the Levant. Garlic has also been unearthed at the royal palace at Knossos.

Garlic is actually mentioned in the Bible. The Israelites bemoaned their inability to get their garlic and onions during the flight out of Egypt to the promised land (again, about 1500 BC). If you want to look it up you'll find it in the Old Testament, in the Book of Numbers, chapter 11, verse 5.

The seafaring peoples of the ancient world, such as the Phoenicians, probably carried garlic in their sea chests, for cooking and healing. This is the most likely route by which garlic was spread from the Middle East into Iberia (Spain) and Southern Gaul and eventually into northern Europe, including perhaps the British Isles.

GARLIC IN ANCIENT GREECE

Together with China and Egypt, Greece was a true powerhouse of learning, accumulated written knowledge and surprising sophistication. Greece was a civilisation of great wealth and intellectual development. The achievements of Greek thought in the fields of philosophy and medicine are the basis of all subsequent developments in medical science in the west. In many ways, the Greeks can be considered to be the founders of modern medicine.

Perhaps the most famous of the Greek physicians was Hippocrates, who lived in the fifth century BC; his dictum 'Do thou no harm' is the watchword of members of today's medical professions, who still take the 'Hippocratic oath' on beginning practice. To Hippocrates' contribution in observing, recording, collating and systematising knowledge of the natural world must be added that of Aristotle, and Plato. Until the eighteenth century, when modern scientific methodology with its experimental rigour became fully developed, the achievements of Greek natural philosophy were the foundation of all medical theory.

Hippocrates recommended garlic for poisoned wounds (gangrene), and for bronchial problems such as pneumonia, catarrh and bronchitis itself. The use of garlic was widespread in ancient Greece and was not without profound religious significance. Garlic appears in the literature, such as Homer's *Iliad*, in which the 'sacred moly' (as Homer calls it) has magical and sacred properties. Garlic

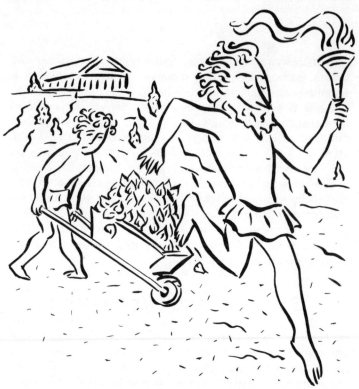

Greek athletic champions knew the benefits of garlic!

appears in the writings of Plato and Aristotle, as well as featuring in temple rites and initiation ceremonies for novitiates preparing to enter the priestly classes. But above all, garlic was favoured as the food of athletes preparing for the great Games.

Garlic was believed to promote stamina and endurance as well as giving energy and super-human strength. We now know that garlic greatly assists in cleansing the respiratory tract and 'thinning' the blood. Consumed regularly, it is highly probable that garlic thus increases the supply of nutrients to the muscle tissue, whilst also speeding up the removal of by-products of energy production, such as lactic acid. This chemical is responsible for cramp and tiredness in the muscle and thus affects performance perhaps more than any other factor. But that's not all. Garlic may well have a mild vaso-dilating effect – it increases the size of veins and arteries – together with 'thinner' blood this will allow a greater supply of strength-giving oxygen to course through the circulatory system.

So Greek athletes obviously had some foundation for their faith in garlic as the food of winners. Garlic also achieved its initial reputation as an aphrodisiac in Greece, but it is to the Romans that we go for the true story of Garlic's reputation for enhancing masculine virility!

THE ROMANS AND GARLIC

The Romans gained their extensive knowledge of garlic's medicinal virtues from the Greeks and Egyptians and it is clear that the magical herb played an important role in the Roman diet and Roman medicine.

While Rome conquered Greece militarily, it is often said that the Romans themselves were conquered by Greek learning and culture. The Romans adopted Greek knowledge of medicine wholesale, and their most important physicians tended to be of Greek nationality, such as Galen, who taught and lectured on herbalism in Rome and was physician to the emperor Marcus Aurelius. The Romans had long been exposed to the discoveries of the Greeks about garlic, therefore. Although some of their cures sound preposterous, there was a sophisticated theory behind them, and a grain of medical truth can often be discerned in what they prescribed.

For boils, carbuncles and abscesses, for example, the Romans mixed powdered garlic with goose grease and ashes from the fire. Whilst this sounds horrendously messy, it is in fact extremely practical. The ashes would abrade the wound and clean out purulent material, whilst the grease would ensure that the site was constantly exposed to the antibiotic qualities of the pulverised garlic. The chances are, we now think, that this remedy would work quickly and efficiently as we know that garlic is a really powerful agent against bacterial infection.

Despite the Romans' reputation for high standards of public health and hygiene, life for the majority would still have been full of the dangers of infections and food poisoning that inevitably follow from conditions of squalor and poverty. Can you imagine the number of gastric upsets that there must have been in those times? Food hygiene was geared simply to prevent food going observably rotten, and garlic, vinegar and salt-petre were widely used to preserve meats and vegetables. There was little personal hygiene for the poor in terms of regular bathing and of course no antibiotics. So plagues and fevers must have been endemic and to gain any resistance to them, you had to contract them and live through the experience! Plants such as garlic must have been worth their weight in gold. In the hands of charlatans, such plants could exert effects and produce cures that would appear miraculous to an untravelled and illiterate peasantry and the idea that garlic was magic would be prevalent amongst the poorer classes.

The story of garlic in the British Isles also begins with the Romans. The invasion of Julius Caesar and his armies was almost certainly responsible for introducing garlic as both a food and medicine to Britain. Those of us who truly love garlic should perhaps thank a chap called Dioscorides, who, although a Greek by birth, was chief physician to the invading Roman forces. Together with Galen, Dioscorides was a major influence on the future progress of medicine in Europe.

Dioscorides had charge of the health of the legions; in all things the Romans were methodical and Dioscorides was responsible for planning and implementing the diet of his soldiers. Garlic was an important staple of their food. Indeed, an expression of the times was 'May you not eat garlic', in other words, 'I hope you don't get called up'! Knowing that Britain was a land of cold and mists, with vast tracts of fen and marsh, Dioscorides would have been aware of the health risks to his troops from fevers, colds and other diseases. So he undertook a great propaganda offensive to ensure that his charges would regard garlic in a completely new light: he persuaded them that garlic was an aphrodisiac, and the Roman Army chewed garlic like there was no tomorrow! There is another side to this story, because the Romans also believed that garlic gave stamina and strength. The forced marches that the legions could undertake were legendary: a distance of forty miles over uncharted rough terrains in one day was not uncommon and here the Romans used garlic as a regular addition to diet.

Diseases such as typhus, cholera and even leprosy would have been rife in the countryside and fevers and diarrhoea would have been the lot of every adult since infancy. Yet garlic could help to reduce fevers, kill intestinal bacteria, clean out infections of the lungs and respiratory tract and deal with internal parasites and skin infections. So it is the

Romans we must thank for bringing garlic to our cold and inhospitable islands.

MEDIEVAL EUROPE

With the decline of Roman political power in the west, much of the heritage of Greek and Roman culture and knowledge was lost. This was a period of great political upheaval and massive population movements, in the midst of which the Church, and especially monasteries and convents, did its best to preserve what was left of the medicinal learning it inherited.

From around AD 350, up until AD 900, garlic all but vanishes from the records. Lovingly cultivated in the medicinal herb gardens of the monasteries, however, it was still around. These are the times when wild garlic was probably used for ailments in humans and certainly used to treat animals for conditions like scours (mastitis) and as a wormer.

The eleventh-century *Physica* of St Hildegard of Bingen specifically mentions garlic as remedy against jaundice. In the sixteenth century, with the growth of medical herbalism across Europe, we find garlic once again both in supply and in general favour. Such luminaries as Paracelsus and Lonicerus, two sixteenth-century herbalists, recommended garlic against poisonings and flatulence, as well as for colic, chills and worms. We also have Sir John Harington's famous verse published in *The English Doctor* in 1607:

> *Sith Garlicke then hath power to save from death,*
> *Bear with it though it make unsavoury breathe,*
> *And scorne not Garlicke like some that thinke,*
> *It only makes men winke and drinke and stinke.*

There are many recorded anecdotes from these times in which garlic's reputation verges on the miraculous. During the fourteenth to seventeenth centuries, the bubonic plague raged repeatedly across Europe killing millions of people. Whole villages were wiped out in weeks; in many English villages today we can see that the church is situated outside the village, whereas usually it would have been the centre of local life. This is a sure sign that the plague came that way: the houses of the dead clustered around the church

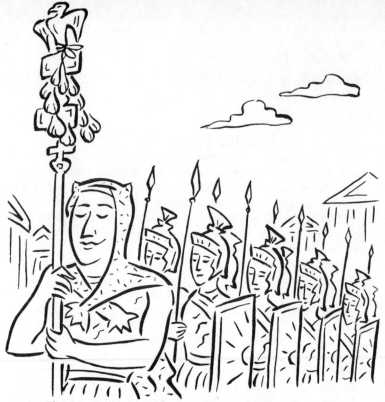

The Roman army's success owed much to garlic (page 16).

were burned to the ground and new houses built a safe distance away, leaving the church isolated from the new construction. You can see such manifestations of the plagues in Suffolk in particular.

To go back to garlic: in France, in 1721 we hear of four thieves who were made to enter the houses of plague victims and load their dead bodies on to carts for transit to the mass graves or plague pits. These four appeared to be immune from catching the plague and survived unscathed despite this practice being deemed a punishment from which they would never return alive. Their secret appeared to be drinking a wine vinegar in which they regularly included a fresh supply of crushed garlic! The particular brew is still available and is known as *vinaigre des quatre voleurs* or 'Four Thieves' Vinegar'.

But that's not all. In Chester is a house with a cellar called now 'God's Providence House'. During the height of the seventeenth-century outbreak of the plague, garlic was stored in the cellars. The entire occupants of this particular property survived the pestilence unscathed, due, it is believed, to the presence of the aroma of crushed garlic – which is a potent anti-bacterial agent. Garlic became accepted as of great value in helping to ward off such diseases and was even used to disinfect the plague pits towards the end of the epidemic.

The best-known traditional belief about garlic, of course, is that it will deter vampires, and in a curious way there is some sense in this! When you eat garlic regularly, its sulphur compounds appear in the lungs and on the skin. Molecules of sulphur are actually excreted from pores, and though you won't notice them, biting insects will. This is an excellent way to be protected against gnat and mosquito bites, and so the peasants who knew this had some reason for thinking that garlic would be efficacious against more deadly and frightening, flying, biting creatures, like vampires!

At the end of the eighteenth century garlic began to vanish from favour in this country – certainly in culinary circles. The German-born Hanoverian kings considered garlic a food fit only for peasants, and it was not to be tolerated at Court. There was no change during the Victorian era. Even Mrs Beeton proposed that persons of taste would use garlic only sparingly and then just to rub the salad bowl!

Garlic made its medical presence felt again during the First World War. It was extensively used by the Russian armies to cure and prevent gangrene. Minced garlic would be applied on a bandage of dried sphagnum moss to suppurating wounds, in many cases avoiding the need for amputation. During the Second World War, garlic was used both to prevent gangrene and for scourges such as typhus and dysentery. Indeed, it achieved the nickname of 'Russian penicillin' for its sterling services.

GARLIC'S DECLINE

Garlic's decline as a medicinal standby was not just due to its unfashionable odour but rather to the advent of drug-based medicines. With the first true antibiotics – the sulfa drugs and subsequently penicillin – old-fashioned country cures based on hedgerow and garden plants fell out of favour. The reasons for this are quite straightforward: firstly it was impossible to know, with traditional medicines, whether what you were using was harmful, especially in the long term; secondly it was hard to prove the value of these cures;

and finally, self-medication for apparently mild symptoms could leave undiscovered other underlying and more serious conditions. If you needed treatment, you should see a doctor!

Scientific methods of analysis and testing were permitting researchers, for the first time, to investigate and identify the precise ingredient in plant material which produced an observable medicinal effect. Increasingly sophisticated understanding of chemistry then allowed them to replicate synthetically that same active material. Having done this, they could provide medicines which gave a precise, measured dose of that identified material to patients. In other words, the hit and miss of herbal medicine had been removed. Commercially, this new regime could also ensure that some of these plant-originated materials could be patented – that is, owned by one company and thus protected against competitive pressures. This gave yet more power to the growing pharmaceutical industry, who rightly claimed such protection as a reward for the work they had invested in their new drug. As new generations have grown up in an increasingly rational, scientific and technological world, traditional knowledge like herbalism came to seem irrational, superstitious and perhaps even dangerous. Medication and health were entrusted firmly to the professionals, and with the growth of a 'cradle to grave' health service it seemed as though traditional herbal medicines might die out completely. This is far from being the case, however: the last couple of decades have seen a vast increase in interest in herbalism, and garlic is at the forefront of this trend.

HERBAL MEDICINE TODAY

The escape of powerful and very dangerous drugs such as thalidomide through the safety net of the rigorous testing procedures demanded in modern times has caused us to be wary of new drug treatments. In addition, there has been a growth in the interest in all things natural and traditional, and a falling-off of faith in 'scientific' fixes for all our problems. The climate of opinion is now much more receptive to the idea that there is much of value to be found in the lore and learning of past generations. We also feel ill-at-ease with complex drug treatments whose purpose and results we don't understand, and look to herbal medicines –

where our problems do not seem to be life-threatening or serious – to help us with ailments that we feel we can and should deal with ourselves.

The growth of sales of garlic, ginseng and evening primrose oil – not to mention royal jelly – is phenomenal. Although not a herbal medicine, cod liver oil is certainly a traditional one and we now know that this natural, safe substance can be of major benefit in the treatment of rheumatism and arthritis, as well as ensuring that, in this sunless land, our body stores of Vitamin D are naturally and easily topped up.

Garlic itself has a Product Licence under the Medicines Act, which allows it to claim that it is valuable in relieving symptoms of colds and influenza such as catarrh and troublesome coughing. In other words garlic is a recognised medicine: after 5000 years it has gained legitimate official recognition in the high-tech world of the 1990s!

Of course 'natural' or herbal medicine has not been ignored by the pharmaceutical industry. Did you know that over 70 per cent of the medicines that you buy in the pharmacy or that are prescribed have their origins in the active principles of plants? This includes aspirin, senna, codeine, digitalis, many antibiotics and anti-fungals, vitamins originally isolated from plants, and, to bring us right up-to-date, rosy periwinkle extract, which is used successfully in childhood leukaemia. This is why there is a last-ditch search going on in threatened areas of the world's forests to gather and preserve unknown and untested exotic plants, to review their chemistry for the next breakthroughs in life-threatening diseases such as cancer.

So plants have played a most significant role in medicine historically and will continue to be the basis of most important medical advances into the future. Garlic is in the forefront of this trend in medical research. Its historically documented benefits are now being proved to be founded in fact, as scientists across the globe investigate garlic and find that it measures up to the challenge of modern scientific review quite magnificently. You can find out more about this in subsequent chapters of this book.

2

Garlic for a long and healthy life

GARLIC AND HEART DISEASE

If you really are curious about garlic and what it can do for your general health, and particularly that of your heart, you need to know a little about what makes both your heart and your body tick.

Heart disease is the major killer in the United Kingdom – some 26 per cent of all deaths occur from this epidemic slayer. It's not just men who die – and die prematurely – over a third of these deaths are amongst women. Although a few people have a pre-determined genetic disposition to heart disease, most of us get to our first heart attack through one thing – poor dietary discipline: we consume far too much fat. Smoking and stress can often tip the balance, ensuring that cardio-vascular disease is the inevitable outcome of a diet rich in animal fats.

WHAT IS HEART DISEASE?

The sign of heart disease is the building-up on the walls of our arteries of a progressively thickening layer of fatty material, which can eventually block the transit of blood. This gradual 'furring-up' of the arteries is known as 'atherosclerosis'. It is progressive and the first streaks of 'atheroma' or deposits of fatty material can often be seen even in the very young. Over time, such deposits can solidify, making the whole area of the artery rigid and inflexible. This is the condition known as 'hardened arteries'.

A hardened artery is fragile and very liable to damage. If the arterial wall is damaged, bleeding will occur and this activates the blood's clotting mechanism, in which a particular kind of blood cell called a 'platelet' is involved. In a normally healthy person, platelets perform a beneficial function as they cause the blood to clot and stop us bleeding to death. In a heart disease sufferer, however, the danger is that platelets will form a patch that could detach itself at a later stage and become lodged in a narrower part of the artery, restricting the blood supply. The restriction of

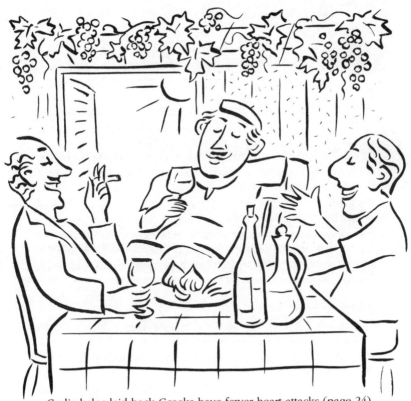

Garlic helps laid-back Greeks have fewer heart attacks (page 24).

the blood supply can cause all manner of complications in the limbs, such as loss of muscle use and of feeling; the most important effect, however, is that in the main arterial supply lines to the heart muscles, such blockages cause the classical heart attack. Here the restriction of the blood supply, with its valuable burden of oxygen and nutrients, damages the heart muscle very quickly and it is this damage which can cause the action of the heart to go seriously awry or to stop completely. If the blood supply to the brain is stopped through congested arteries or from a clot which blocks the arterial bore, then this is known as a stroke.

WHAT CAUSES HEART DISEASE?

It is necessary to understand what causes the condition we know as 'hardened arteries', and what role is played by the three 'baddies' – poor diet, smoking and stress – if we are to understand why garlic could play such an important role in protecting heart health.

The Buck, Donner and Simpson study

A few years ago an important study[1] was conducted at the University of Western Ontario to determine which factors were most important in a population's predisposition to heart disease – and, conversely, which factors were not. The countries the researchers examined included Belgium, Chile, Costa Rica, France, Greece, West Germany, Italy, Japan, Mexico, Portugal, Singapore, Spain and Switzerland. All of these countries report mortality statistics by causes of death; they also keep statistics on consumption per head of cigarettes, different types of wine and dietary staples, including onions and garlic. The researchers looked at the figures for all of these intakes over the years 1972 to 1975 and attempted to find a correlation between them and death caused by heart disease.

The results

The results of this research were startlingly clear in their implications for the relation between diet and heart disease. The correlation between a high intake of saturated fat and a high incidence of heart disease was striking, as was that for smoking. On the other hand, higher levels of garlic and onion consumption coincided with lower levels of heart disease in all the groups examined. Alcohol didn't seem to make much difference. The final conclusions of this massive exercise were that the higher the consumption of garlic and onions within a population, then the lower the incidence of and mortality from heart disease.

This bears out a striking north/south bias in Europe too. Until recently Finland was the heart attack capital of the world, but dietary advice sponsored by the government and regular check-ups have now moved the Finnish male way down the league in just ten short years. It's we, here in the United Kingdom, who top the polls at present, and, in general, it is in the north that the incidence of heart disease is at its highest. Go down to sunny Greece. Cardio-vascular disease is minimal there, yet they eat their fat-laden menus with relish and smoke their heads off! But they also love their peppers, onions, garlic and spices. The same is true of Spain and Italy. More and more the finger points towards a regular consumption of garlic and, to a lesser extent, onions too as one of the ways of keeping heart disease at bay.

THE FATS STORY

Now it's known that diet is one of the main causes of heart disease, many people are prepared to change their diet in the interests of keeping healthy. The first thing to do is to move away from the typical fatty western diet – but it can be very hard to know which fats to avoid.

Saturated, unsaturated and polyunsaturated Fats

Saturated fats will increase the levels of cholesterol in the blood. This type of fat comes mainly from dietary sources such as meat and dairy products. The fats in fish, especially the oily varieties, in chicken and turkey and in most vegetable oils are largely unsaturated. (And in poultry, most of the fat is contained in the skin which can be left uneaten if you wish.) These fats do not contribute to the presence of blood cholesterol. Vegetable oils also contain a group of fats known as polyunsaturates. These are believed by some to be actually beneficial to cardio-vascular health. But, just to complicate matters, a recent school of thought suggests that the so-called mono-unsaturated oils are even better for us. These are found particularly in ground nut oils and olive oils. But there are yet other factors in the fats story to be considered.

THE CHOLESTEROL STORY

In any discussion about heart health the word 'cholesterol' invariably crops up. But seldom do we find an explanation of the true role of cholesterol and just how essential it is to life. We can't survive without it, but too much of it, on the other hand, is one of the root causes of the life-threatening cardio-vascular disease.

What cholesterol is and isn't

Cholesterol is a fatty substance that is present in certain foods, mainly – though not exclusively – in fatty foods such as animal meats. Small amounts of it are essential for making and maintaining cell membranes and for making natural hormones which are the regulators of body behaviour. Yet you do not need to eat cholesterol-rich foods such as fatty meats and dairy products in order to get your daily quota of this chemical. Your liver (which actually *makes* cholesterol for you) can use many other foods to ensure you get your necessary supplies. If you were to cut out all cholesterol-rich

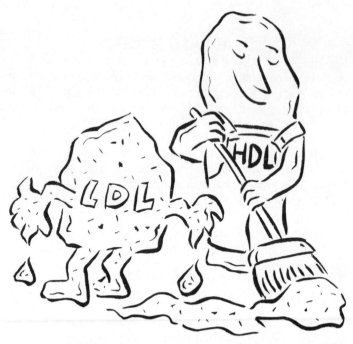

HDL 'caretakers' clean up excess cholesterol!

food from your diet from today onwards, you would lower the cholesterol content of your body by about 15 per cent. It might not sound much, but that 15 per cent might make all the difference between the healthy functioning of your body and the development of a life-threatening disorder! High cholesterol in your blood will almost certainly lead to a narrowing of the arteries as a direct result of the deposition of atheromas, which I have previously described. So including only small quantities of cholesterol in you diet will lower your blood cholesterol levels by an appreciable percentage, with a proportional lowering of the risks of cardio-vascular disease. But it's not quite so simple as that. If it were then we could all guarantee that heart disease would be a thing of the past.

LDLs AND HDLs

It isn't enough just to state that we should cut down our consumption of cholesterol. We also need to know why it can cause problems and in order to understand this we have to know how cholesterol travels around the body and what it actually does. Cholesterol is carried around the bloodstream by complex little pieces of protein called lipoproteins. The main lipoprotein is Low Density Lipoprotein (LDL). 'Lipo' just means fat. LDLs are made in the liver, from where they cruise around the bloodstream carrying cholesterol. But where do they deliver it to? Along the walls of the arteries, as well as in other parts of the body, are cholesterol-receptive sites which, through a complex system of chemical messages, talk to the LDLs and get them to drop their parcels of cholesterol. If you've over-indulged in some cream cakes, and had double eggs and bacon with fried bread on the side, these little sites will be overwhelmed – there will not be sufficient of them to handle the vastly increased LDLs carrying the extra cholesterol produced by your dietary excesses. So the LDLs simply dump it in the wrong places, for example the walls of your arteries. And so a gradual furring-up begins and that's the start of cardio-vascular disease.

Fortunately there's another type of protein, known as a High Density Lipoprotein (HDL). This is manufactured by the liver and acts as a sort of arterial cleanser – it moves around your bloodstream looking for dumped cholesterol, which it collects and delivers back to the liver, ready for disposal. It would seem as if this would provide a natural balance, but what happens when you have high LDLs and low HDLs? Cholesterol material is deposited where it's not wanted and there are insufficient cleansers to pick it up and take it back. Result – atherosclerosis.

Getting the best balance between HDLs and LDLs

Oily fish and garlic both appear to affect the way in which dietary fats are handled by the liver. Even after meals high in saturated fat, garlic seems to regulate the liver's production of HDL/LDLs beneficially in favour of HDLs. In the next chapter we will discuss studies on the effects of garlic that have produced evidence of this and have demonstrated the important fact that garlic will, very quickly after it has been eaten, reduce the stickiness of blood platelets to a much safer level – another valuable benefit when considering how to keep your heart and circulation healthy. Most interestingly, it seems that garlic is unique in providing both of these important benefits.

WHAT YOU CAN DO FOR YOUR HEART

The objectives for heart health are relatively simple – even if difficult to achieve without considerable will power!

1. Cut down on saturated animal fats in your diet and substitute low-fat alternatives, such as polyunsaturated fat spreads, low-fat cheeses and skimmed milk. If you eat meat then make sure it's chicken or very lean meat, and grill it rather than frying it.

Very recent research based on findings from the Eskimo diet have shown that a pound or so of really oily fish every week can do wonders in preventing the arteries from becoming clogged, so eat fish such as mackerel and herring frequently.

2. Stop smoking. It makes your blood platelets stickier, although the reason for this is not fully understood.

3. Find ways of alleviating stress, such as taking up relaxation classes or yoga. Yoga is a system of simple but very beneficial exercising, and you don't have to be a contortionist to do it. Yoga can help you feel serene and peaceful if you take it seriously and it only takes a few minutes each day.

4. Keep your heart muscles in good condition. You don't need to be an Olympic athlete to do this. A good *brisk* walk that gets you out of breath two to three times a week is a real tonic – aim for a couple of miles each time. This will help to get your resting pulse rate down by increasing the strength of the heart muscle and improving lung action; the heart therefore needs to work less hard and consequently beats more slowly. A low resting pulse rate is a sign of good heart health.

5. Take everything in moderation. Cut down on coffee and tea and take only the occasional glass of wine. Don't binge, especially on chocolate or any caffeine-rich foods or drinks. Caffeine is a stimulant and can over-stimulate your heart.

6. Take *garlic* every day, raw, cooked or as a supplement.

GARLIC AND BUGS AND BACTERIA

Any discussion of the value of garlic to human health would be only half complete if there were no mention of garlic's potent activity against most of the disease-causing organisms known as bacteria.

Bacteria are microscopic living creatures that are a miracle of both function and adaptability. They can multiply at prodigious speeds and can evolve to build up resistance against antibiotics which once would have killed them. They live in the air, soil, water, our homes and, of course, inside our bodies. Those that live within us are generally beneficial and coexist with us in a state of symbiosis. Without them we should probably die, as they carry out some very important functions, especially in the gastro-intestinal tract. They also fight unwelcome invading bacteria in a similar way to that in which white blood cells fight off intruders in the bloodstream. In a healthy body the 'good' bacteria live in a state of balance with the 'bad' bacteria that ensures a basic physical harmony. The 'bad' bacteria are called pathogenic bacteria, or pathogens for short. They populate our nasal linings, throats, mucous membranes, lungs and parts of our gastro-intestinal tracts. While we are fit and healthy they are kept in check by our own body defences, but when our resistance is lowered they can multiply to such an extent that they cause problems.

It is not only the bacteria themselves that cause ill health, however, but the byproducts they excrete – bacterial toxins (poisons) – and the more of them there are, the more poisons they put into our systems. These toxins are simply the result of the bacteria producing energy and waste products. Both bacteria and their toxins cause diseases.

GARLIC – A POTENT ANTI-BACTERIAL

Garlic kills bacteria – even some of the nastiest and potentially life-threatening forms. Scientists have proved this by growing bacteria and then adding garlic extracts to the established colonies; garlic very quickly kills the thriving bugs and prevents further growth. But this is laboratory work. What happens inside the human body and how do we know that garlic is effective in real life? The way in which garlic eventually exits from the body gives some important clues.

GARLIC'S ROUTE TO EXCRETION

Everything you eat or drink is acted upon by the body in many complex ways. In these actions, time and body heat are important factors. It will take between 12 and 36 hours for most materials to work their way through your system to final excretion, and during this process your body will take valuable components that it needs for repair, growth and energy from these materials. In this process, which we call digestion, the body will apply its own chemicals such as enzymes and acids to nutritional materials and change them into forms, called metabolites, which are able to produce the absorbable and useful compounds that it needs. Garlic metabolites are the important substances as far as garlic's anti-bacterial action is concerned.

Once the important constituents of food have been removed through the digestive processes, the body eliminates unwanted materials through the kidneys, liver, lungs and skin. In considering the function of garlic, the last two assume great importance. Compounds produced from garlic are actively present in the lungs as part of the excretion process and they are able to exert an anti-bacterial effect in lung tissue, thus guarding against bronchitis and other infections. These compounds are also excreted heavily by the mucous membranes, which again explains why garlic is so valuable in helping to clear up catarrh and sinusitis. Garlic is also expelled through the skin in micro-quantities of sulphur compounds that are present in sebum – the material excreted through our sweat glands. You can't smell them, but fleas, gnats and mosquitoes can and will avoid you like the plague!

GARLIC IN THE BLOODSTREAM

This presence of garlic in various areas of the body tells us something else important; to reach these areas, garlic compounds must have been carried there via the blood supply. In other words, once you have eaten garlic it is converted into absorbable sulphur compounds which are then carried in the blood as both nutrients and medicinal

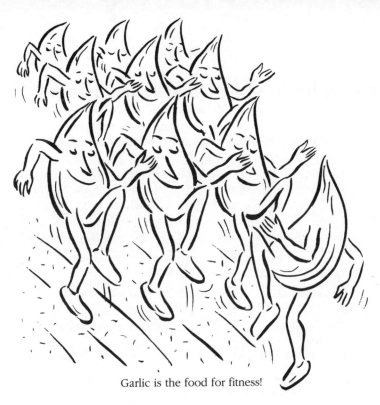

Garlic is the food for fitness!

materials throughout the body. This explains how garlic is able to deal with internal parasites as well as many skin problems.

GARLIC ON THE BREATH

Since garlic compounds are excreted partly though your lungs, the smell of garlic will also appear on your breath. There's little you can do about this apart from sucking a mint! Chewing fresh parsley or cardamom seeds will mask the smell initially, but not when the garlic begins to be excreted through the lungs. It used to be thought that the smell of garlic in the mouth arose from odours in the stomach, but even with the advent of capsules and tablets, where the active garlic material is not released until it is lower down in the small intestines, garlic's odour on the breath is still evident in some people. This may seem a considerable drawback, but were garlic not excreted through the lungs we should lose the protection it gives us against chest problems. People will notice garlic on your breath, but as you add garlic increasingly to your diet your body will become accustomed to it and the smell will become less evident.

WHAT ELSE CAN GARLIC DO?

Because garlic breaks down into a number of compounds (see chapter 3) it is able to function as a whole family of medicines and thus cure a number of ailments. The following list will give you a very good idea of the conditions for which garlic has been used with success historically. In appendix A (page 89) you will find a summary of some of the most interesting recent scientific research that, in quite a few of these health-problem areas, is showing that there may be reason to take garlic's ancient reputation seriously.

Arthritis
Arteriosclerosis
Asthma
Athlete's Foot
Bronchitis
Cancer (certain kinds only)

Catarrh
Cholera
Common cold
Constipation
Dandruff
Diabetes
Dog bites
Oedema (excess bodily fluids)
Dyspepsia
Dysentery
Eye burns
Gangrene
Hypertension (high blood pressure)

Influenza
Flatulence
Jaundice
Lead poisoning
Leprosy
Lip and mouth disorders
Malaria
Measles
Meningitis
Haemorrhoids
Rheumatism
Ringworm
Scorpion stings
Septic poisoning
Smallpox
Tuberculosis
Typhoid
Tetanus

3

How garlic works – an easy garlic chemistry lesson

We know that garlic has been used for centuries as a remedy in many areas of human health. But oral and written history from past generations isn't considered to be proof of a cure in this scientific age. Today, facts have to be proved beyond doubt, and this means undertaking what is known as a clinical trial.

This, simply put, is a controlled experiment carried out under ideal conditions and constantly monitored to ensure that no external factors distort the final results. As part of the trial, pre-determined levels of the substance to be tested are given, according to a strict regime, to a defined group of subjects – in the case of garlic trials, human beings. Measurements of the effects of the substance given are then very carefully made and the results plotted and analysed. By controlling every aspect of the trial, the testers aim to ensure that their results will be valid according to the most rigorous scientific standards.

CONSTRUCTING A SIMPLE TRIAL

Let us review the procedures of a simple trial. A group of volunteers are put on an identical diet, which does not contain any ingredients that might interfere with results. For example, ginger would be banned because it can affect platelet stickiness results. Certain drugs would also be disallowed. The volunteers are all given exactly the same quantities of food.

Next, the group is divided into sub-groups, each with the same number of subjects. Let us use three groups for this hypothetical trial. Group 1 will continue with the group diet and not take any garlic. Group 2 will continue with the group diet but will have a predetermined level of garlic also included – it might be raw, cooked or in the form of tablets or capsules. Group 3 will continue with the group diet but will be given food or capsules which, although they may smell of garlic, will not actually have any active garlic materials present.

Group 1 will be called the Control Group, Group 2 will be called the Active Group, and Group 3 will be called the Placebo Group. A 'placebo' – literally 'I will do no harm' is simply a device to see if making people believe that they are on an active therapy actually produces results.

Before starting on the various diets above, each member of the groups will have his or her blood-fat levels and platelet stickiness levels measured. This is essential to show the normal levels of activity in the individual's blood. It therefore becomes a yardstick against which to measure the changes that may occur within each of the groups as the trial progresses.

The trial may be for a week, a month or even longer. Blood-fat and platelet stickiness measurements are taken at regular intervals and at the end of the trial. The diet is then stopped and the subjects return to their normal dietary habits.

But that may not be the end of it. Further samples and measurements may be taken a week or so after the subjects are back on their normal diets, to see if the changes noted

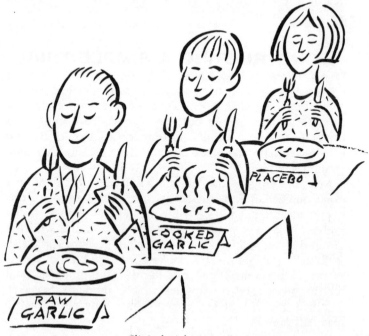

Clinical trial 'victims'!

in the trial period have been maintained or if there is a movement back to the results seen in the measurements taken prior to the trial commencing.

What I have described so far would be a fairly straightforward and uncomplicated trial. Trials can be much more complex, however. For example, a trial might also test the effects of garlic taken at the same time as eating a meal rich in saturated fats. Testers would establish a fourth group, whose basic diet was high in saturated fats and who took garlic as did the Active group; they might even have a fifth group whose fat-rich diet was given with a placebo.

Such clinical trials can be very complicated. In addition, groups can be switched around, for example, the subjects might spend half the time of the trial in one group and half in another. However they are designed, the objective of a clinical trial is to test whether the substances on trial have any effect or are inactive.

Over the last 30 years or so, garlic has been regularly used in trials on both humans and animals, particularly in the area of its possible actions on blood-fats and the platelet adhesiveness mechanism. The majority of results obtained by these trials have been very supportive of garlic's actions in these two important areas of cardio-vascular health. Before we go into scientific proofs, however, we need to know a lot more about what happens to garlic when it is eaten or taken as a tablet or capsule. And, perhaps even more important, what happens to the miracle molecule, allicin.

ALLICIN

A clove of garlic does not have any smell while it is still intact, but as soon as it is crushed or cut it gives off a pungent odour. This is because there are two separate substances in each of the millions of cells that make up each clove, which, as long as the clove remains intact, remain apart. Once the clove is damaged they are brought into contact with one another and a material called allicin is produced.

Allicin has a very short life and begins to biodegrade from the moment it is made. If the garlic is put into a refrigerator it will still contain allicin a few days later, but if it is left at room temperature for the same length of time, analysis will show that all or most of the allicin has gone.

As allicin breaks down it takes oxygen from the air and begins to turn into sulphur-rich chemicals. In due course it will produce over 70 different organo-sulphur materials, some of which are thought to be stable and thus able to remain formed and complete. Others continue to break down into basic sulphur compounds, which so far appear to have little beneficial value.

Allicin itself is no longer thought to be the active material in garlic; it is the stable organo-sulphur materials that are believed to be medicinal, and it is because there are so many of them that garlic has a remedial action in so many different diseases.

So what happens to allicin when you eat raw garlic – and when you cook it? And what happens when you take a garlic tablet or capsule?

EATING RAW GARLIC

When you chew a clove of raw garlic, you actually create allicin in your mouth. When you swallow it, it moves down your gullet and into your stomach. Here it meets with concentrated hydrochloric acid which starts the process of digestion. When the stomach empties (an involuntary action that you won't know has happened) the garlic material moves into the duodenum, where it is acted upon by digestive enzymes. Eventually it arrives in the small intestine, where the process of absorption into your blood stream finally takes place.

We know that allicin is unstable above a very low temperature, yet your body will quickly raise its temperature to around 98°F (37°) and it will also be exposed to acids and enzymes. The clove of garlic you originally chewed will not present itself in your intestines until some hours later and by this stage it is unlikely that any allicin is left; it will have commenced the process of breakdown almost as soon as you created it in your mouth.

So what is present? The answer is that at this stage we don't really know with certainty, but we do have some interesting clues.

EATING COOKED GARLIC

The good news here is that boiled and fried garlic appear to have the same beneficial effects on the cardio-vascular system as the same weight of raw garlic. What is interesting is that this also supports the story that allicin is not the active material. Frying chopped garlic or boiling cloves of garlic have produced good results in clinical trials in direct comparison with raw materials. Yet there is not the remotest possibility that any allicin could survive in the high temperatures used in cooking.

THE ACTIVE MATERIALS IN GARLIC

The Japanese have synthetically produced[2] one of the compounds that arises as a direct result of the breakdown of allicin – Methyl Allyl Trisulphide (MATS) – and tested it thoroughly. MATS appears to be very effective in quickly reducing the tendency of blood platelets to clot. Other compounds, such as Di Allyl Disulphide (the major component of garlic's essential oils) have also been proposed as active materials, as have several other sulphur-bearing compounds which are the direct result of allicin breakdown.

ESSENTIAL OIL

When we look at essential oil of garlic, we have the final part of the argument that allicin is not the active principle in garlic.

Essential oil of garlic is prepared by steam distillation. In this process, steam is passed through mashed garlic. The steam vapourises the oil and carries it, in suspension, to a condenser. Here the steam turns back to water and oil. The oil floats on the surface of the water and is run off for refining. The heat of the steam and the time taken for the process breaks down all of the allicin, so that none can be found in the oil. But what can be found and measured precisely is a whole range of sulphur compounds such as MATS, which are the direct effect of the conversion of allicin by heating.

Scientists agree

Recently several interesting statements have been made by world-ranking scientists about allicin and garlic. The first is that allicin is not the active substance in garlic – it is only the starter material. The second is that the action of garlic is now believed to come from oil-based materials in garlic and not the water-soluble ones. One trial actually tested the water in which garlic had been boiled against the boiled garlic itself – and showed clearly that the water was totally inactive.

THE CLINICAL TRIALS

The results of several hundreds of trials from all around the world where garlic has been tested on humans have been published. We are going to look at the results of testing raw garlic, cooked garlic and garlic in health products. Because of the very wide range and the vast number of papers which have been published, I have selected two or three relating to each type of garlic mentioned above and attempted to present their findings in an easily digestible form.

RAW GARLIC COMPARED TO FRIED GARLIC

In 1981, Doctors Chutani and Bordia of the Drug Research Centre at Tagore Medical College in India produced a paper[5] which compared the effects of raw and fried garlic in 20 patients who already had a long history of heart disease. All patients had evidence of arterial scarring because they had previously suffered from blood-clotting. The purpose of the trial was to discover the degree of activity of these two forms of garlic on fibrinolytic activity in humans. Briefly, if you increase the blood's fibrinolytic activity you reduce its tendency to form clots (by reducing its overall stickiness) and also increase its ability to dissolve existing clots. Success in this area is an important and valuable attribute in overall cardio-vascular health.

Patients had blood samples taken prior to the exercise and these were analysed to measure fibrinolytic activity. All patients continued with their normal diets during the trial and they were told not to make any changes to them which might affect final results.

Garlic cloves were given at 0.5 g per 1 kg of body weight – around 30 g (or 12 cloves) for a 60 kg (around 9 stone) person. This was either mashed in butter (raw) or fried in butter. The person who analysed the subsequent blood measurements did not know which patient had been given which form of garlic – a most important precaution to ensure no bias creeps in! A further group of patients who did not receive garlic acted as a control, so the requirements of a properly conducted trial were fulfilled.

The trial was further divided into two segments, the first of which was a short-term or 'acute' study; a later stage lasted up to six weeks.

Results

I quote from the authors' summary of findings, firstly from the shorter, acute study.

> '...Fibrinolytic activity increased by 72 per cent and 63 per cent within 6 hours of administration of raw or fried garlic respectively. The elevated levels were maintained for up to 12 hours.'

For the longer term study the results were even better.

> '...it showed a sustained increase, rising to 84.8 per cent at the end of the 28th day when raw garlic was administered – similarly with fried garlic the rise was 72 per cent.'

The authors also came to several other important conclusions. There is a small loss in potency when garlic is fried but the loss is not significant. Further, the garlic has a very fast effect, achieving its peak some six hours after it is eaten, and this effect is maintained if garlic is taken in the diet on a regular basis. Their final paragraph is well worth quoting too:

> 'The present study clearly demonstrates that garlic, whether eaten fried or raw, may prove to be an important dietary measure for everyday use by persons who appear to be predisposed to thrombotic complications. *Thus the general belief that garlic would lose most of its effect by cooking is wrong and even after it has lost its acrid smell* [through cooking] *garlic still retains its beneficial effect on fibrinolytic activity.*' [Author's italics]

As a general note, the percentage enhancement of fibrinolytic activity shown by the above trials is remarkable by any standards, and clearly shows that garlic is of great value in controlling this primary aspect of cardio-vascular health, and doing so with absolute safety.

RAW GARLIC COMPARED TO BOILED GARLIC

This trial by Sharma and colleagues was reported in the *Indian Journal of Nutritional Dietetics* in 1976[4]. It set out deliberately to increase the fat-loading of the trial subjects' blood by adding large quantities of butter to their diet. This was then challenged by both raw and boiled garlic, both to see the effects on blood-fat levels and to see which was the most effective form of garlic for such a challenge.

Twelve healthy volunteers below the age of 40 were used; these fasted for 12 hours before the experiment began. After giving an initial blood sample to review starting blood-fat levels, each took an identical fatty meal consisting of 100 g of butter fat with four slices of bread. New blood samples were then taken after two and four hour intervals to measure the increase in blood-fat levels. On the next day this procedure was repeated in identical fashion, but this time 50 g of a crushed paste of raw garlic was added to the meal. On the third day, 50 g of boiled garlic cloves were given with the fatty meal. On day four only the water in which the garlic had been boiled was given. Blood-fat measurements were taken at regular intervals to measure the effectiveness of each treatment in suppressing the automatic rise in blood-fats which occurs after consuming saturated fats such as butter.

Results

I quote from the author's summary of findings:

> '...the data indicates that ingestion of a butter fat meal increased the total serum cholesterol [the fat loading found in the bloodstream], by a mean [average] of 38 per cent after four hours...When garlic was administered with a fatty meal, both forms of it, raw and boiled, were found to prevent the increase in levels of total serum

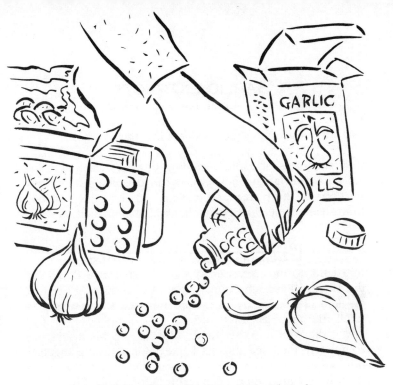

Garlic preparations also show good trial results.

cholesterol....When the water in which garlic cloves were boiled was given with a fatty meal, no cholesterol-lowering effect was noted.'

There are many such trials reported in the extensive literature on garlic which show quite conclusively that regular daily use of garlic as a cooked vegetable can assist in reducing the blood's ability to clot, while also beneficially changing the elevated blood-fat loading which occurs after a meal rich in saturated fats.

These results make you look at such traditional meals as what we now call a 'Ploughman's Lunch' – a huge chunk of the saturated fat known as cheese, accompanied by an equally large, fresh onion. The onion has similar effects to the garlic, but you have to eat much more of it than you do of garlic. Did our forbears know that onions would help to abate the effects of cheese which, being a rich source of protein is a beneficial food, but is very high in fat? Probably they based their choice on the compatibility of the two tastes, but this is still a striking example of the uncanny way that nature arranges things.

GARLIC EXTRACTS

We've looked briefly at both raw and cooked garlic; now let us discuss garlic extracts, as these are what many people use as a way of getting garlic goodness into their bodies.

Again, there are hundreds of papers which look at many different forms of garlic, including powders, extracts using solvents such as alcohol (which can dissolve out the oily fractions of the plant), and essential oils of garlic resulting from steam distillation. Let us start with essential oils.

ESSENTIAL OIL IN TRIALS

In a letter to the *Lancet* in April 1981[5], Dr David Boullin of the Medical Research Council Clinical Pharmacology Unit at the Radcliffe Infirmary in Oxford reported the results of a small trial amongst three subjects who simply ate 10 g of raw garlic with no other food. According to his results this completely inhibited platelet aggregation (sticking together or clotting) within an hour of eating, despite his also trying to induce aggregation chemically beforehand. This effect was still present some three hours later. But the important conclusion of Dr Boullin's experiment was his proposal that this resulted from Methyl Allyl Trisulphide which, we have already seen, is a constituent of essential oil of garlic (at between 5 and 12 $\frac{1}{2}$ per cent of the total oil).

In January of the same year, three members of the Nippon University School of Medicine had also submitted a letter to the *Lancet*[2]. They advised that they had isolated a component of garlic oil which they had identified as Methyl Allyl Trisulphide and had gone on to synthesise this into a 98 per cent pure product. This was tested for its inhibitory effects against platelet aggregation, which they used certain chemicals to induce deliberately. Its effects were found to be exceedingly powerful in only minute concentrations in blood plasma. Their final comments were :

> 'The effects of Di Allyl Disulphide (the major constituent of garlic oil at some 60 per cent of total volume) was less than one tenth of that of Methyl Allyl Trisulphide. The application of MATS as an antithrombotic agent is now being studied.'

These letter extracts are important, because they show the direction in which researchers are moving. There are key active elements hidden in the components of garlic which are produced through the digestive process and through cooking. Scientists with increasingly sophisticated and rigorous methods of analysis can individually isolate even tiny amounts of complex compounds and test them for effectiveness both in the laboratory as well as in humans and animals. The identification, extraction and synthesis of MATS is a good example of how this can be done.

In 1986, a paper appeared in the *Journal of Traditional Chinese Medicine* entitled 'The Effect of Essential Oil of Garlic on Hyperlipaemia and Platelet Aggregation'[6]. (Hyperlipaemia means high blood-fat levels.) This was an analysis of some 308 patients and was presented by the Cooperative Group for Essential Oil of Garlic from the Zheijang Institute.

In any terms this was a major study in which subjects were classified into groups according to their fasting blood cholesterol levels and also to their history in terms of previous heart and arterial diseases.

In Group 1, 51 per cent had a history of high blood pressure and 21 per cent had coronary heart disease or had presented symptoms of it. Group 2 included 34 patients with very high blood-fat levels and an enhanced overall platelet aggregation rate. Each group contained both males and females.

Capsules of essential oil of garlic prepared from 25 g of raw plant were prepared for taking at two capsules per day (50 mg total per day). The course of the treatment was to be 30 days for Group 1 and 20 days for Group 2. Prior to the start an exhaustive battery of tests were done, including: electrocardiograms (a complete review of the action of the heart done electronically); blood and urine examination; liver-function testing and blood-fats measurements. The patients kept to their normal diets and took no other medicines during the trials.

Results

The results from this trial are truly excellent and clearly show the benefits of daily consumption of garlic.

Group 1 comprised 274 patients with fasting blood cholesterol levels that were greatly above average. After treatment with the essential oil capsules at two per day for 30 days, all blood-fat levels showed dramatic decreases of around 20 per cent or more. When considering this drop, remember that these patients had a history of higher than average blood-fat levels and that any downwards movement was of great significance in terms of enhanced future heart and arterial health.

Group 2 exhibited similar tendencies, with a considerable reuction of blood-fat content to within normal levels.

In 85 cases in Group 1, a rise in HDLs was noted in the area of 10 per cent; in 60 cases from Group 1 a 43 per cent reduction was achieved in 'plasma fibrinogen', which exists in the bloodstream primarily for the purpose of producing clots. Subsequent attempts to induce clotting of patients' blood after taking the garlic course showed that the aggregation or clumping/clotting rate had dropped by around 30 per cent.

Many other measurements were included in this thorough review of garlic oil and the author's concluding comments are worth noting:

> 'In brief, essential oil of garlic definitely reduces serum lipids, plasma fibrinogen, platelet aggregation rate and blood pressure while the oil raises the serum HDL and promotes fibrinolytic [clot-dissolving] activity. Since it acts on the many aspects associated with atherogenesis [the formation of fat deposits in arteries], its probable multi-action therapeutic effect on cardio-vascular disease merits due attention.'

POWDERED GARLIC IN TRIALS

Recent trials[7] of powdered garlic material have confirmed that garlic is also effective in this form, but material has to be very carefully prepared to keep the allicin-forming materials separate from one another in the final powder before it is made into tablets. This is done by carefully slicing garlic to prevent as much as possible of the allicin-forming substances from coming together to create allicin. The sliced garlic is then gently dried and made into powder, and then into tablets. The tablets are not dissolved until they have exited from the stomach, thus forming allicin and its

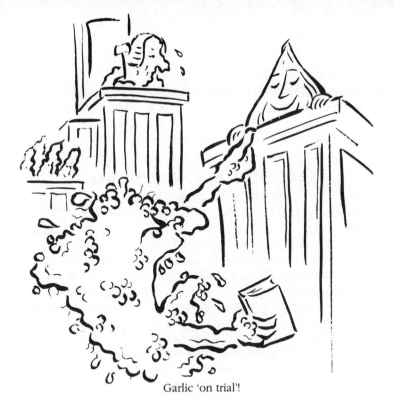

Garlic 'on trial'!

byproducts further down the digestive tract. As, however, the allicin thus produced still has to be converted into absorbable materials that we know are active, powders are another way of providing the activity of raw garlic without too much of the smell.

Powders do have one drawback, however – they are equivalent to only three times their weight in raw plant materials. Therefore, you have to take quite a lot of powder to represent a significant quantity of raw garlic.

Most of the trials done on raw garlic range from around 12 g per day up to 50 g. My own view is that two to three cloves a day (about 8–9 g) are a useful and healthy dose for those whose diet is normally balanced in terms of fat intake. To achieve this with powders, you would need to take around 3 g of dried material. If you convert this into tablets of around 100 mg each, then you need to take 30 of these daily to get your raw garlic equivalent. Recent trials[7], however, suggest that quite low doses of 6–12 tablets a day can help to reduce platelet stickiness and cholesterol levels.

This is another area where essential oils score. With extraction rates in the region of 1500–2000 parts of plant to one part of oil, plus the benefits of refining and blending to achieve high levels of active materials such as MATS, much higher doses of garlic equivalent can be taken in very small quantities of essential oils. These smaller doses can easily be carried in a single daily capsule with no difficulty.

GARLIC'S ANTI-BACTERIAL ACTION ON TRIAL

This is a very difficult area in which to carry out trials in humans. Do you give a human control a particular disease to see if garlic cures him or her? Of course not. But what we can do is grow organisms in the laboratory and then challenge them with garlic to see if they survive or die.

Many animal trials have also been undertaken, in which it is known precisely what the problem organism is that is causing a particular infection. In chickens, dogs and horses, garlic has been widely used historically for bacterial infections such as mastitis, lung disorders and infections of the gut. But it is in the microbiological laboratory that the true power of garlic can be seen.

All laboratory work is of necessity carried out in artificial conditions and only surmise can then relate any findings to how such test materials might work when applied to a human being. Nevertheless, it is well worth considering the scientists' findings from the vast number of trials against harmful organisms, both bacterial and fungal, which have been carried out in the laboratory.

The most potent action undoubtedly arises from allicin itself which is exceedingly powerful when tested against practically all pathogenic bacteria and indeed fungal organisms. But we know that in real life, allicin only exists for a short time, so how do we explain the activity of garlic against problem infections of the respiratory tract, gut and skin?

At present we simply don't know enough to explain garlic's unique ability, but there are some clues.

Prior to the advent of life-saving penicillins which themselves were originally derived from living moulds, a class of antibiotic substances called sulfa-drugs did sterling service in the Second World War. Their activity was based on sulphur compounds and it is this element in garlic which is at the bottom of its long history as a potent antiseptic and bactericide.

Tuberculosis

This disease was once a major killer. The bacterium that causes it is particularly resistant to treatment, implanting itself so deeply in lung tissue that it is hard to get at. Garlic's excretion through the lungs means that its sulphur-bearing materials are present at cellular level and are all pervading, thus ensuring that the whole area of infected tissue is exposed to potential treatment. Garlic cures for TB were often extremely successful, but the treatment itself could be drastic – although perfectly safe. Patients would take tonics made from crushed garlic in milk and olive oil. They would have external poultices of garlic crushed into a blanket of oil-soaked lint applied to the chest and back and, as if that were not enough, they would regularly inhale the fumes of garlic which had been freshly crushed into a nasal steam bath to which boiling water had been added. Such treatments were a full frontal assault on the disease, aimed to get garlic into the body through the digestive, respiratory and blood circulation routes. But they did work and there are many recorded instances of success against this dreadful disease.

Cholera, typhoid and dysentery

These diseases are caused by organisms which can readily become resistant to antibiotic therapy. They are all life-threatening and are still endemic in many countries today. Garlic had achieved a magnificent reputation historically against these disorders and its action was confirmed in laboratory tests against the precise classes of bacteria responsible for these diseases in the last century.

Yet garlic has another benefit which is vitally important. Antibiotics have the ability to kill all bacteria in the human system, including some that are beneficial. This can create a whole new range of problems. After a short while, harmful bacteria may colonise the vacant sites left by the beneficial bacteria which have been removed. It is not uncommon for patients on antibiotic therapy to find that another infection, such as candida, takes over. A sore mouth or throat can often be the sign that a secondary infection of another type has occurred after a course of antibiotics.

Garlic's actions appear to be somewhat different. While the harmful bacteria may be successfully eradicated by garlic, the useful bacteria do not appear to be eliminated.

They simply defend themselves by changing their state into an inactive one, waiting for the time when they can again commence to grow. They can therefore take over their old site after garlic has done its work.

This is not all. Bacteria cannot become resistant to the actions of garlic, whereas some types of bacteria do become resistant to antibiotics in time. This inability to become resistant to garlic's powers suggests that it is not just one particular fraction of garlic that is operating but rather a multitude of sulphur-bearing compounds. In other words, if one part of garlic doesn't get you then another part will. But we're still not much nearer to finding out exactly what parts of garlic work against bacteria, except in the laboratory – and this is not real life.

Nevertheless, present-day laboratory work suggests that garlic is at least as effective as most of the normally used antibiotics when tested directly against bugs grown artificially. The acid test is really how garlic can benefit you and under what conditions. This is covered in chapter 4, but undoubtedly garlic can help in a long list of infections of the gut, skin and respiratory tract. Even better, garlic is a potent preventative agent against a whole range of such problems if taken every day. This protective way of using garlic is, in my opinion, the best way to get your garlic goodness. As a rule of thumb, garlic is believed to have one tenth of the power of an equivalent weight of penicillin.

GARLIC AND VIRUSES

Garlic certainly works against verrucae, which are caused by a virus infection. Tape a thin slice of fresh garlic over a verruca with a sticking plaster, change it for a fresh slice each day, and within a week to ten days the verruca will come away. Certain warts will also respond to this kind of treatment (but do not take action against warts yourself – see your doctor if these worry you). Even the humble corn will respond to the above treatment, but this is probably due to an acidic reaction which is keratolytic – the garlic material eating away dead or dying skin and allowing the corn to come away from the healthy tissue. Verrucae, however, are too deep for this to be the explanation of garlic's action on these conditions.

But does garlic work against such viruses as influenza? According to the letters we receive at the Garlic Research Bureau, the answer is a definite YES! How it works we do not know, but it may be something to do with garlic's ability to produce a warming and drying action generally, to stimulate the blood flow and thus to produce additional energy. Such an increase in overall metabolism may well confer a general strengthening of the overall immune system. The answer is to try it for yourself the next time you fall prey to winter ailments.

Coughs and colds

As we know, some garlic oil products have a full product licence for the symptoms of coughs and colds. Garlic has gained this new official credibility mainly through its action in the lungs and sinuses. In the former it guards against secondary infections which can arise from the mucosal

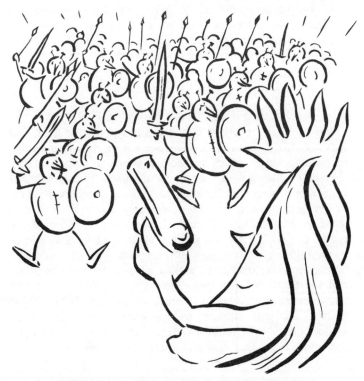

Garlic 'zaps' the bugs that cause coughs and colds!

secretions of a head cold, some of which will end up in your lung cavity. While your resistance is low from colds or 'flu you are open to secondary bacterial infection of lung tissue, which means that bronchitis is a potential problem whenever you get a really nasty cold. Taking garlic during such an episode makes excellent sense as it can often prevent such a possibilty.

Many older people have tried taking garlic right through the winter and have experienced no chest problems at all, whereas formerly they would spend the winter months wheezing and coughing with sore chests and aching lungs. No official trials have ever been carried out in this area, because it is too difficult to design such a trial, so we have to rely on anecdotal evidence and on the increasing numbers of people who wouldn't be without their garlic every winter.

For catarrh, garlic really is a must. Raw garlic will fix even the most intransigent choking mucus within a few hours only. It appears to do this by drying up the secretions and by killing the infections that are causing the mucus to be made by the sinal passages. But a head cold is a viral infection, not a bacterial one – so is garlic an anti-viral agent too?

GARLIC AND CANCERS

This is a highly charged and necessarily emotive area. Just let's say that there is some evidence for the proposition that garlic may have activity for certain kinds of tumour under certain conditions. It was certainly used historically for cancer and a recent Chinese study (see appendix A, page 92) suggests that garlic taken regularly in food can confer some protection against stomach cancers and those of the colon. But such trials and any accompanying stories must be viewed through a very powerful scientific pair of spectacles. Garlic may be useful as a part of diet to help regulate general health but we cannot jump to any conclusions that it will ever be the answer to curing all cancers. What we do know is that garlic appears to help keep the immune system – the body's own natural defence mechanism – in good condition; more than that it is impossible to say.

4

Time for action – getting garlic goodness into your life

There are many practical ways in which you can start including garlic in your life with very little problem even if you are worried about the odoriferous consequences! Ultimately, the best garlic must be the garlic you grow yourself – in your own garden or even in a sunny windowbox.

GROWING YOUR OWN GARLIC

If you have tried growing garlic before without much success, don't be discouraged. There are a few easy requirements for growing really superb garlic and if you follow these simple instructions you should experience no problems.

Firstly, get the best seed cloves you can find. The individual clove is taken from the outside of a freshly bought bulb and will eventually grow (rather like a shallot) into a complete new bulb. This type of culinary garlic is known as *Allium sativum.*

Secondly, find a sunny location. A south-facing plot or window box is the best. This is vital since garlic needs long hours of good light to grow successfully.

Thirdly, garlic loves a light, sandy soil. You may add a little bonemeal and a sprinkling of sulphate of potash (which is rich in sulphurs) to give your garlic that extra boost in terms of flavour and strength. Remember that it is the sulphur content of garlic that gives it its important health benefits. Garlic plants take sulphur from the soil as they grow, so the more sulphur there is in the soil the greater the curative properties of the garlic. I suggest a mixture of 1 part of good-quality general compost and 1 part of washed sharp sand.

PREPARING YOUR SEED CLOVES

Buy a couple of firm, reasonably large bulbs from your greengrocer or supermarket, strip off the outer paper-like membrane and carefully break off the individual cloves.

Only use the cloves from the outside of the bulb and be careful not to break each clove's individual skin. Carefully inspect each clove, only keeping those that are absolutely perfect with no blemishes. Make sure also that they are quite firm to the touch.

PREPARING THE GROWING MEDIUM

Garlic likes a reasonable depth of soil, so if you're using a window box or pot then a depth of 15 cm (6 inches) is the minimum for a good root system on which the health and life of your plants will depend. If you are going to use a garden bed the soil should be well-dug and worked, then sieved to a reasonably fine tilth. If the soil is heavy and waterlogged add peat and rotted compost to lighten it, plus plenty of washed sharp sand to give good drainage. Garlic abhors waterlogged soil and will not develop properly unless drainage is really excellent. Work some bonemeal into the soil at about 12 g per sq m ($\frac{1}{2}$ oz per sq yd) for a long-term fertilising effect and sprinkle a little sulphate of potash on to the area, forking this in to the top 10–15 cm (4–6 inches). The site should be exposed to the sun from early in the morning until dusk, so a south-facing position is really a must.

PLANTING

November is the ideal time for planting so that the root system can develop over the winter months. The young shoots will then get a feast of sunshine throughout the spring and summer seasons. Make sure you position each clove in the soil with the pointed end up and the base at a depth of around 4 cm ($1\frac{1}{2}$ inches). Plant the cloves at 15 cm (6-inch) intervals. Gently firm down the soil and then water in well.

Growing garlic requires little attention other than keeping free of weeds and watering frequently – but don't drench it. Just keep the soil moist; little and often is the best rule.

HARVESTING

When the plants flower you should remove the flower heads as this helps to conserve energy, and probably flavour, in the root. Around July the tops will begin to wilt and brown

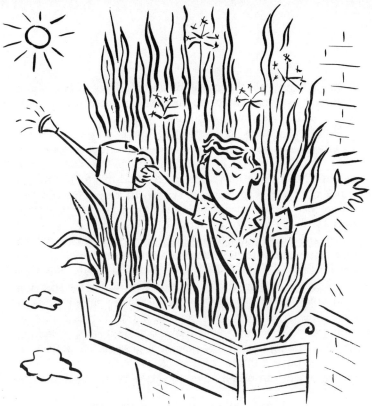

'Growing your own' gives good results!

off and during August the bulbs will be ready for harvesting. Take care when lifting garlic – despite appearances it is quite a tender plant and if bruised will quickly blemish. Carefully wash and dry each root and then hang up by the leaves in a cool dry and airy room or shed. (Sun drying is best but not always practicable in our climate.)

Once the bulbs are fully dried they can be kept in a cool place until required. Keep them away from other produce which may itself rot and subsequently cause your garlic to rot too. Garlic for relatively immediate use can be stored in the refrigerator quite safely for a few weeks. Your newly-grown garlic will last until the start of the next growing season and possibly through until the middle of the next season – around 18 months in all if stored properly.

GARLIC IN THE GARDEN

Garlic has a variety of uses in the garden, from companion planting to insecticidal and anti-fungal applications. It has long been grown with rose bushes, since the vapour arising from its leaves will keep aphids and mildews at bay – and rumour has it that garlic grown next to a rose will actually enhance the sweetness of the rose's perfume.

However, garlic's most effective use is as an insecticide and fungicide. Here's how to make up an effective solution.

Take 100 g (4 oz) of garlic and peel the skin off the cloves. Crush these into a fine paste. Add this to 150 ml ($^1/_4$ pint) of vegetable oil and stir well. Keep this in the refrigerator for 24 hours, stirring occasionally. The vegetable oil will slowly absorb the active oils from the cloves. Strain the mixture and add 900 ml ($1^1/_2$ pints) of water to which you have added a few squirts of washing-up liquid to ensure the oil is emulsified throughout the water. Stir well and keep cool. This can be diluted with water for spraying at around 50:1 and is effective against many garden pests. It also clings to foliage and, as it dries out, leaves a minute sulphur-based residue which is a deterrent to sap-sucking and leaf-cutting insects. For persistent pests, dilute at 25:1

If you have trouble with bank or field voles, or with moles, which can ruin a flower bed or a lawn respectively in a few hours, place crushed garlic bulbs in the entrances of their burrows. The sulphurs leach out into the surrounding soil and, while not harmful to plants, emit their powerful vapours for many weeks, acting as a deterrent to rodents.

An anti-mosquito agent

Garlic oil has been used regularly in many countries to eradicate the mosquito in its breeding sites. The life-cycle of a mosquito involves a larval stage, during which it infests shallow stretches of water, before the mature insect emerges. Garlic oil in very low concentrations incorporated with a detergent agent is sprayed on to the surface of the water. This appears to affect the way in which the developing larvae put together certain protein structures and they die before maturity.

Garlic's effectiveness as an insecticide in the domestic garden may be based on the same process.

GARLIC SUPPLIERS

Getting high quality seed corms is a matter of your own judgement when it comes to obtaining them from your local store. However, there are commercial garlic growers in the

United Kingdom who have achieved an enviable reputation for producing garlic of excellent quality. Quite the largest grower of culinary garlic is Colin Boswell, of Mersley Farms in the Isle of Wight. His farms are situated in one of the most picturesque valleys on the island. The rich, red, alluvial soils are of a fine, porous sand and loam mixture, free-draining and able to hold the sun's heat. But the real merits of the Isle of Wight lie in its long hours of sunlight – just the thing for growing really fat and flavourful garlic. The garlic Colin Boswell cultivates is of French origin and has been developed by him through progressive selection to produce garlic which is fat and juicy while being both firm in texture and full of flavour. He now grows some 150 tonnes per annum, all of which quickly vanishes into the cooking pots and frying-pans of Britain. Colin also supplies seed corms to those who wish to start growing their own, together with a leaflet with full cultural instructions on how to get the very best quality crops. If you'd like a supply of ready to plant top quality seed corms then write to Mersley Farms, on the Isle of Wight (see appendix B).

THE NEWCHURCH GARLIC FESTIVAL

Each year, usually during August, Colin and his father Martin organise and run the biggest garlic festival in Europe. The festival is held on a Sunday and around 30,000 visitors are attracted, with all proceeds going to a worthwhile charity. There are marching bands, flying and motorcycle displays plus all the fun of the fair! If you can get across to Newchurch for this splendid day you will not be disappointed. Colin Boswell will send details of the next festival date with your order.

THE GILROY GARLIC FESTIVAL

This is held in Gilroy, California, and is the biggest garlic festival in the world. Nobody can do it like the Americans can – hundreds of thousands of visitors come from all around the world for this garlic extravaganza. All the food and a lot of the drink is spiced liberally with garlic, including ice cream and jello. If you like garlic this is the place to be. The US Tourist Office (see appendix B) can give you details if you feel that this is an opportunity not to be missed.

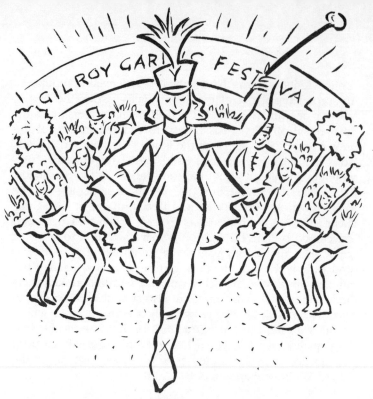

The Gilroy Garlic Festival, California.

GARLIC AND YOUR PETS

Garlic is one of the best all-round medicines for the simpler ailments of a wide range of pets. The commercial world is fast becoming aware of the power of garlic and numerous products are now available to get garlic's goodness into your pet on a regular basis.

Much of what we now see in herbal medication of animals we owe to the Romanies, who prized garlic above all herbs for curing illness in both themselves and their animals. Garlic remedies abounded, generally mixed with other field and woodland herbs, for a whole range of animal health problems.

Today, research into treating animals with garlic is going on apace. Even the chicken is the subject of research to see the effects of garlic on the composition of the saturated fats in egg yolks, and garlic is being tested on chickens infected with salmonella[8].

PIGEONS AND CAGED BIRDS

Garlic is really important to the pigeon-racing fraternity. It helps improve speed and general stamina, as well as keeping the feathers free from fungal infestations and skin disorders. Ask any keen racing man if he uses garlic and the answer will be that he wouldn't be without it! As a general treatment for caged birds, a tiny amount of crushed garlic paste can be shaken up with their seed and then removed. The seed will have taken up sufficient oil for a beneficial effect to be obtained. This is ideal at moulting time, when the general condition of the skin is poor, and is also useful whenever the bird is relatively inactive or generally in poor health. It is a cheap but very effective treatment, and quite safe.

DOGS

Along with pure cod liver oils, garlic is probably one of the most beneficial additions to your dog's daily diet that you can possibly make. As garlic is an effective worming agent, it will ensure that any eggs from tape and thread worm are safely eliminated and that the animal's digestive processes are kept properly functioning and in good health. As happens in humans, some of garlic's sulphurs are excreted through the skin and this will keep your dog free from problems such as mange and infestation by ticks and fleas. Garlic also helps to keep down 'doggy' smells, especially those arising from the coat and the breath.

Just like humans, dogs can suffer from viral infections and chestiness. Garlic helps to ward off such infections and to keep the animal generally healthy. Lameness and poor circulation are also known to have been beneficially affected by regular garlic administration.

Give a regular daily dose either of garlic oil pearles or tablets. One 0.66 mg garlic oil capsule is sufficient for small breeds; give two for medium-sized breeds and a one-a-day pearle for larger animals.

CATS

Cats do not normally like odoriferous materials, particularly those such as pine oil and orange oil that are highly aromatic. Yet they will take garlic in the form of tablets or capsules. For most cats the benefits are the same as for dogs. Give one tablet or capsule daily, with some liquid such as milk or water to follow.

HORSES AND PONIES

Both the French and the Irish have known about the value of garlic in maintaining horse health for centuries. The French particularly will treat clots on joints with garlic poultices and include fresh garlic or garlic oil in feed. For problems such as colic and croup, garlic is a winner every time. Signal success with severe problems such as sweet itch have also been achieved with regular administration of garlic. Coughing and bronchitic conditions will be eased by the use of fresh garlic ground into a paste and added to honey. A sensible daily dose for a pony would be four to five cloves daily, while a large hunter will need some twelve to fifteen cloves daily. Again, garlic will help to keep the coat in good order, sweeten the breath and regulate the digestion. Many an old hack has been brought back to life using garlic's restorative powers.

GARLIC PRODUCTS IN THE SHOPS

Garlic products are very big business. From small beginnings around ten years ago, garlic product sales are now worth some £10,000,000 at over-the-counter prices, and they continue to grow at a prodigious rate as more and more people realise that a regular consumption of garlic will keep them healthy with only a small effect on their pockets. But the people who must really take the credit for the garlic's growing success are the owners of hundreds of local health food shops, who in past years promoted garlic despite the fact that its use as a medicine was regarded with derision.

It's probable that around a million people in the United Kingdom use garlic as a preventative against winter ailments, for stomach upsets or simply as a daily tonic. But a new group of users is now joining them – those whose GPs have said that garlic might well be good for them. These are people with high blood-fats or a history of heart and arterial problems. So garlic is booming – but what sort of garlic should you take?

TABLETS

We have already discussed the new ways of making powders to conserve their 'allicin-forming' potential. The higher quality products use this method as it is the best way to ensure that the finished product is as near to fresh raw garlic as it is possible to get with a dried extract. The higher the quantity of allicin-making materials in a given weight of raw garlic or in the resultant powders, the more effective the garlic is going to be.

POWDERS

Powders claim to be three times more potent than the same weight of raw fresh garlic. This yield of one part of powder to three parts of original plant is the usual ratio we expect when dried plant material is made into a powder. But the limitation is that you need to take a lot of powder as tablets to get a meaningful dose of raw garlic equivalent. One 100 mg tablet is equal to around 330 mg of plant material. Therefore, to get the equivalent of 3 g of plant (a medium-sized clove) you need to take nine tablets. The tablets could be made bigger but many people cannot swallow tablets easily, so the present size of 100 mg of powder per tablet is most practicable.

Most of the trials using raw garlic feature daily garlic intake from 12–50 g and tablets would have to be consumed in considerable numbers to achieve these daily levels. However, recent trials[7] have suggested that 6–12 tablets a day may well have a preventative effect against cardio-vascular degeneration, although this relatively low level (the equivalent of 1.8 g of raw garlic) is well below that used in most trials.

In this context it is interesting to note the German authorities' requirements for garlic products. They will permit manufacturers to claim that their products guard against arterial ageing if they contain the raw plant equivalent of 4 g of raw garlic in a daily dose.

Many people find tablets the most convenient way of taking garlic and an ongoing programme of trial work will eventually show conclusively how effective they really are.

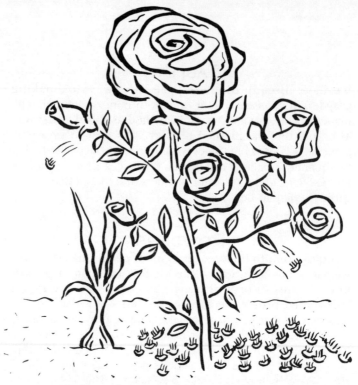

Garlic can be a powerful insecticide (page 54).

ESSENTIAL OILS

Essential oil is my personal choice. I have used it for over twenty years for conditions such as diarrhoea and gastric upset, tooth abscesses and coughs and colds.

Essential oil is a very potent expression of garlic's strength, being distilled from between 1500 and 2000 times its own weight of raw plant. The process of extraction converts the allicin which is made when the raw bulbs are first mashed into the distilling vessel. The resultant oil can then be analysed for a whole spectrum of organo-sulphur compounds, some of which are quite stable and will survive the digestive system largely unchanged and ready for action when they are finally absorbed into the bloodstream.

GARLIC PEARLES

Essential oil of garlic is supplied in soft gelatine capsules or pearles. The oil is contained in a carrier oil such as soy bean oil, since it is far too potent to take on its own and only small quantities are required to give high clove equivalents.

For instance, 1 mg of oil is equal to around 1.5–2 g of garlic (one small clove). Therefore, to get the equivalent of 4 small cloves (12 g of garlic) you need only 6–8 mg of oil. Such high doses could be put into a single capsule with ease. This is an obvious route for future development, to permit high doses of oil to be taken regularly.

As with tablets, there is good evidence that oils are effective in helping to ensure cardio-vascular health and also in warding off infections.

DEODORISED PRODUCTS

Until recently the process of deodorisation was considered by some scientists to remove completely the antibiotic and cardio-vascular benefits of garlic; now opinions are changing. Although the organo-sulphur compounds present in conventional garlic products are unlikely to be found in the odourless products, the original garlic sulphur content is still in the materials used to make them.

One way in which such materials are made is by mashing raw garlic, putting this mash into a tank under a pressure 'blanket' of nitrogen gas which traps the vapours in the mash, then adding special yeasts which 'digest' these volatile sulphur fumes until they have all been removed. Once this has been accomplished, the yeasts expire and the mash is prepared as a paste for incorporation into a capsule or tablet. None of the original sulphurs contained in the raw garlic starter material has escaped and the sulphur content of the mash will still be there – but in a different chemical form.

There are many other ways in which deodorising can be carried out and the Japanese particularly have spent much time and money in producing and testing deodorised materials. In my opinion, such products are worth considering and the people who use them certainly testify to their effectiveness.

GARLIC AND CHILDREN

Garlic is safe for the majority of people but children are a special case. Although garlic-eating mothers-to-be have smelt garlic's all-pervading presence on the first breaths of their newborn children, you must be careful when considering garlic for the very young. This is not because it is harmful, but rather that the digestive system and the overall metabolism of the infant takes some while to develop fully and garlic can cause gastric upset if taken at an early age. Consequently, garlic tablets and capsules should not be given to children under six years old. Children up to ten should receive only half of the adult dose of lower potency products (three tablets daily at 100 mg or one oil capsule at 0.66 mg oil content). Above ten years old there should be no problems with the adult dose, but do stick to the pack instructions. While garlic is one of the few medicines where more means better, do not apply this rule to children.

WHAT KINDS OF GARLIC REALLY WORK?

The really good news is that all forms of garlic offer benefits to the regular user. Whether you take garlic raw, cooked or as a capsule or tablet, it will be good for you. We know this from clinical trials, where all forms of garlic have been tested on humans for conditions as diverse as heart disease and cancer. But we know from other information sources too – letters from users, articles in magazines, from personal experience and especially from the experiences of past generations.

I should like to record some instances of how garlic has helped me. I have always believed that personal experimentation is a good thing, provided always that you have some knowledge of what is wrong with you and that it is not too serious.

I have travelled quite extensively in parts of the world where a bad attack of stomach problems was guaranteed within a few days of arriving, and prior to learning about garlic I would always take a private prescription for a very powerful antibiotic with me. Once I discovered the powers of garlic I decided that the next time I was *in extremis*, I would try a handful of garlic oil pearles and see what happened. I did so and within a few hours I found complete relief and suffered no recurrence of the symptoms. From then on I have always carried my garlic with me whenever going overseas and it has never failed me yet.

Garlic has not just helped with stomach problems in other

countries. On one occasion, after I had eaten two lightly poached eggs, I suffered griping pains in my stomach of worrying intensity. Drawing on my previous experiences, I swallowed ten of the one-a-day garlic oil capsules and within an hour the symptoms had completely subsided. I believe I had probably contracted *Salmonella enteritides* – but I cannot prove it.

A further experiment involved the nagging presence of an abscessed tooth. The pain from this condition can be extreme, but I did not want to take antibiotics as these kill all micro-organisms, including the beneficial ones. So, like the Ancient Egyptians, I thought of garlic. I took a handful of capsules and within two hours the pain had subsided. I kept the offending tooth and the problem has not returned.

TREATING YOURSELF
WITH GARLIC

Before we take a look at the many ways in which you can use garlic for your health, please remember that symptoms of any problems which either persist for more than a few days or which are distressing should be presented to your doctor. This precautionary advice by no means demeans garlic or its capabilities but takes into account the fact that, however well informed we each may be, we are not always equipped to distinguish critically between what may only be a minor problem and what could be a much more serious condition. Bearing this in mind, we will first look at some of the ailments for which fresh garlic can be used. Always keep remedies made from raw garlic refrigerated to protect its active materials from decay.

SORE THROATS AND UPPER
RESPIRATORY TRACT INFECTIONS

Make a garlic syrup by taking six or seven large cloves of garlic and mashing them into a paste. Add six teaspoonfuls of wine vinegar and stir. Leave in the refrigerator for 24 hours to marinate. Warm 50 g (2 oz) of best honey until quite liquid and stir in four teaspoonfuls of lemon juice. When quite cool add this to the garlic paste and again stir well. Keep in a closed jar in the fridge until required. For use for a sore throat, take two teaspoonfuls and retain in the

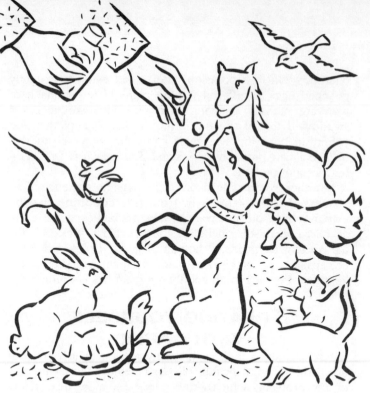

Garlic is good for keeping pets healthy too!

mouth until very liquid. Then gently allow this to trickle down your throat, giving a little gargle now and then to bathe the back of the mouth and tonsils. Repeat three times a day.

For a wheezy cough, take a dessertspoonful of the syrup first thing in the morning and last thing at night. For catarrh take two teaspoonfuls three times a day. This will leave a breath odour but it is extremely effective.

UPSET STOMACH AND DIARRHOEA

Garlic is an excellent and fast-acting remedy for getting your digestive organs back into normal play.

Take three large cloves of garlic and crush them into a paste. Add one dessertspoonful of olive oil and mix well, Slowly add three tablespoonfuls of slightly warmed full cream milk. Stir well and then drink. You may sweeten this with sugar or honey if you wish.

Again this will leave an odour but that is a small price to pay for its effectiveness. If symptoms persist for more than

24 hours consult your doctor. With such problems in infants and young children *always* get medical advice – do not assume that you know what is wrong with them as you could be mistaken.

GARLIC AS A GENERAL TONIC

Take six to eight large cloves of garlic and crush them into a paste. Add four teaspoonfuls of finely chopped parsley and the same quantity of lemon juice. Stir well and keep in the fridge for 24 hours, stirring every three or four hours. Finally, add 250 ml (8 fl oz) of white wine (sweet or dry), stir well and return to the fridge. Take two teaspoonfuls of this mixture twice a day, preferably first thing in the morning and last thing at night. You will have garlic on your breath but you will feel like a million dollars after taking this elixir of life for a week!

MOUTH ULCERS AND FUNGAL INFECTIONS OF THE MOUTH

Mouth ulcers are another medical mystery. They are extremely difficult to treat and again little is known about why and how they occur. This treatment is very effective if you have soreness in the mouth from a fungal infection or ulcers on the gums or soft tissues.

Take two dessertspoonfuls of natural yogurt. Crush three cloves of garlic to a paste and mix thoroughly with the yogurt. Take two teaspoonfuls of this mixture, retaining it in your mouth and swishing it around the affected areas with your tongue. It may sting a little at first but persevere. Keep this up for a few minutes and then spit out the mixture. Repeat three times daily. You will also find some pain relief from this remedy and the condition will normally clear up within four to five days. However, if this is a persistent problem and you have had the condition for more than a week, then please see your dentist – there are many mouth conditions which only he or she can treat.

GARLIC THROUGH THE SKIN

Garlic applied directly to the skin can cause a stinging sensation unless it is accompanied by a soothing material such as milk, honey or oils. Yet it is worth persevering because it is effective against athlete's foot, acne, cuts, bites, stings and skin eruptions such as boils and infected sebaceous cysts, described below.

Many essential oils have the ability to pass through the skin and obtain direct access to the bloodstream after application. This is a most important part of the now increasingly popular practice of aromatherapy. Garlic oil will very quickly gain access to the bloodstream if applied almost anywhere on the body. After just a short time, its odour will appear on the breath too. Indeed, in many Eastern European countries, where eating raw garlic is a way of life to protect people against fierce winters and the diseases that constant cold can bring, small children who refuse to eat raw garlic are given it in a different way. Garlic cloves are crushed into a paste and put into the child's shoes. After even a short time, the unmistakeable odour can be smelt on the child's breath. Garlic's essential oils have been absorbed through the skin of the sole of the foot, have passed through the bloodstream and thus into the lungs – mothers can know for sure that their children have received their dose of garlic and are thus protected against colds and 'flu. If you try this, be warned that on sensitive skin garlic can cause a rash.

ACNE

For acne, at least four or five cloves of garlic should be included in the daily diet. This should be supplemented with a garlic product, either six to twelve tablets or three one-a-day capsules daily. Existing eruptions should be bathed in garlic lotion. Take 250 ml (8 fl oz) of surgical spirit and add to this 12 g (1½ oz) of freshly made garlic paste. Stir well and keep refrigerated. This should be dabbed on regularly. The mixture is a little smelly, but a few weeks only of this treatment will work and the initial odour dies off quite quickly after application. The liquid dries out the skin and helps to unclog blocked pores which will usually quickly become infected. Diet should be controlled to remove refined sugars and all animal fats and dairy products during the treatment period.

ATHLETE'S FOOT

This is a fungal infection which can be both painful and distressing. The remedy again is a simple one. Take two tablespoonfuls of olive oil and add to this four medium cloves of garlic crushed into a paste. Stir well and leave for 24 hours. Apply the oil between the toes three or four times a day. For a quicker result soak cotton wool balls in the oil, squeeze out any surplus and wedge these between the toes. Change this dressing daily. At night continue the treatment, but please do wear socks unless you want the bed to hum with the aroma of garlic.

BITES AND STINGS

Slice a fresh clove of garlic and rub it immediately on to the site of the bite or sting (ensuring first that any sting has been carefully removed).

BOILS AND CYSTS

Take a piece of clean lint and cut it into an oblong about 2.5 × 5 cm (1 × 2 inches). Soak this in olive oil and gently wring out the surplus. Crush a garlic clove finely and anoint one half of the lint with the resultant paste. Fold over the other half of the lint to make the crushed clove into a 2.5 cm (1-inch) square sandwich. Apply this directly over the boil or cyst with sticky tape. Change this dressing daily. This helps to relieve the pain and inflammation and will break down the plug blocking the sebaceous duct very quickly. If you have sensitive skin, apply petroleum jelly round the swelling to ensure that the pad only comes in contact with the erupting head of the infected area.

COLD SORES

These are caused by the herpes virus. Once you have con-tracted the virus you harbour it for life and it manifests itself when you get a little run down. Garlic appears to have an inhibiting effect on cold sores and so does coffee, probably due to its high tannin content. Even if you have suffered from cold sores for years, this little remedy is well worth a try.

Take a level teaspoonful of dried instant coffee and mix to a paste in an equal amount of natural yogurt. Crush two

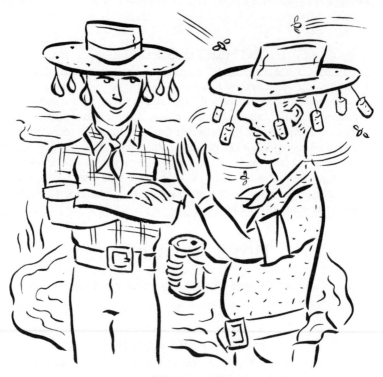

Flying insects (like vampires) hate garlic!

cloves of garlic to a paste and add these to the mixture. Add about a teaspoonful of set honey and enough cornflour to thicken to a creamy paste.

Apply this to the affected area regularly. The mixture will eventually dry out and fall off – simply apply some more. This remedy is not recommended for its cosmetic appearance but it does work if you persevere!

VERRUCAE

Take a fresh clove of garlic and remove a thin slice across the clove with a razor blade or sharp knife. Anoint the unaffected area immediately around the site of the verruca with petroleum jelly so that the garlic will not come into contact with it. Place the garlic on the verucca and hold with sticky tape or a plaster. Apply a fresh slice daily. After a week to ten days the verucca should come away completely. Like herpes, this is a viral complaint and very little is known about how these conditions can be successfully treated. Garlic seems to be one of the very few answers.

Garlic as an insect repellant

If you are an angler or a hiker, or if you just spend a lot of time in woodlands or down by a river, mosquitos and gnats can be a real problem. Regular consumption of garlic is a most effective repellant against such insects; for some reason, the liberation of minute quantities of sulphur in human perspiration effectively deters them from biting. As the perspiration dries out the sulphur is trapped under the minute hairs on the skin surface and is sufficiently strong to warn insects off.

If you do not want to eat garlic for such protection, squeezing a garlic pearle into some petroleum jelly and anointing your arms, face and neck with this will also give excellent results. However, the dietary treatment is preferable since it also protects against the insects that get inside your clothes.

Garlic and protection against food poisoning

We are becoming increasingly aware of the problems imposed by twentieth-century environmental changes and many of these affect us directly. Contaminated food and water, for example, are of great concern to many people and, as we have already seen, garlic can be of help in combating stomach upsets. Its role in keeping us healthy also makes us more resistant to the onset of such ailments. This is discussed more fully in chapter 5.

We have seen that garlic does not appear to harm those beneficial bacteria which live in harmony with us – but it is a death-dealing material against harmful bacteria, especially those which invade the gastro-intestinal tract as a result of eating contaminated foods. Eating garlic will put its powers directly in contact with harmful bacteria in the gut, but because some of garlic's active materials are absorbed into the bloodstream, it also acts within the whole body to give additional protection.

We also know that garlic appears to be able to neutralise some of the effects of the toxins produced by many gut-borne bacteria, as well as eradicating the bacteria themselves.

If you are concerned about eggs and poultry, chilled ready-prepared foods or any other aspect of food hygiene, the simple answer is to take garlic each day.

My way of doing this is to ensure that at least one meal each day includes two or three cloves of garlic – boiled or fried, it adds new zest and flavour to many commonplace dishes. But I also supplement my diet with a commercial garlic product – and here there is a choice of oil-filled capsules (pearles) or tablets. A normal daily dose of these products contains sufficient antibiotic power to give a high level of protection against most food-poisoning bacteria. Remember that once you have made garlic a regular feature of your daily life, your body will contain a much higher level of effective sulphur compounds which will give you around-the-clock protection every single day.

How to take garlic products

As we have discussed, taking an active garlic product means that odour must at some stage be evident on the breath as the active materials in garlic are partly excreted through the lungs. One of the best ways to keep this to a minimum is to be careful about just when you take your chosen products. My advice is always to take them with a little cold water immediately before a meal. Because the garlic will be mixed with food, there will be less likelihood of it causing wind (which can often occur with garlic products when taken by themselves). Also, the passage of food into the digestive tract switches on acid production and thus ensures ready assimilation of the garlic together with your food. This helps to neutralise the effects of any saturated fats in the meal, which is beneficial to the health of your arterial system.

Cooking for health with garlic

Once again, do remember that cooked garlic, that is, both fried and boiled, is very valuable for helping to maintain good health. As a garlic beginner, adding garlic progressively to your own and your family's diet will do nothing but good.

Other important culinary flavourings which complement garlic are oregano, sweet basil and anise. With these three, plus your garlic, you can create mouthwatering dishes in true continental and oriental styles. Again, grow them yourself!

70

GARLIC BREAD

Most people use butter, but any examination of the diets of southern Europe shows clearly that using olive oil as a cooking medium is much healthier for your heart.

Take 2–3 medium-size garlic cloves, 2 tablespoonfuls of best-quality olive oil and 1 stick of french bread. Crush the garlic into a smooth paste in a garlic press. Put this in a cup and add the olive oil. Stir well and leave for a few minutes for the garlic oils to dissolve into the olive oil. Cut the bread into partial slices – slice nearly the whole way through the loaf but not quite. Then prise apart each slice without breaking them off the loaf and coat both surfaces of each slice with the garlic and oil mixture (a pastry brush is best for doing this). Then wrap the loaf in greaseproof paper and pop it in the microwave on Full Power for 1 to 1^1/$_2$ minutes, or wrap it in foil and place in an oven preheated to 180°C, 350°F, Gas Mark 4 and leave for around 10 minutes. I prefer to use the oven as opposed to the quicker microwave as it gives a far better distribution of the garlic's flavour throughout the loaf. Serve immediately, as it should be eaten piping hot. This is a great acompaniment to meat-based soups, or you can simply eat it with a fresh chilled salad.

GARLIC, BACON AND VEGETABLE SOUP

This soup is wholesome and filling and is especially suitable as a winter warmer.

4 rashers back bacon, trimmed
^{1}/$_2$ small green pepper
1 medium-size English onion
1 large garlic clove
1 tablespoon vegetable oil
3 celery sticks
50 g (2 oz) button mushrooms
1 cup shredded spinach
2–3 medium-size carrots
2 tomatoes
2 tablespoons cornflour
chopped fresh oregano or basil, to taste
salt and freshly ground black pepper

Cut the bacon into thin strips, using kitchen scissors. Dice the pepper and onion into 1 cm ($^1/_2$-inch) cubes. Slice the garlic very finely and put the bacon, peppers, garlic and onion into a frying-pan with one teaspoonful of good quality oil and fry gently until golden brown.

Cut the celery, mushrooms, carrots and tomatoes into small pieces and, together with the spinach, season well.

When the bacon, peppers, garlic and onion are cooked, drain off the oil and place them into a large saucepan. Add the other vegetables and 600 ml (1 pint) of water. Mix the cornflour with a little water. Add further water until a milky consistency is obtained. Add this to the saucepan too.

Gently bring to the boil, stirring occasionally, then turn down to simmer. Cook for 30–45 minutes. Add herbs such as oregano or basil to taste and check the seasoning.

Strain off the bacon and vegetables to leave a creamy soup or process the whole mixture in the blender and reheat before serving. This is especially good with Garlic Bread.

Serves 1–2

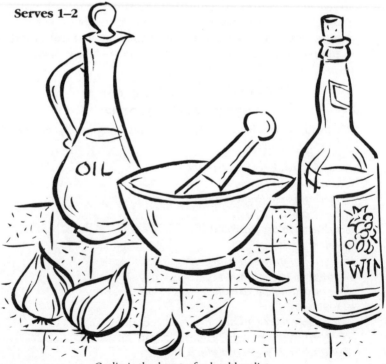

Garlic is the heart of a healthy diet.

PEPPING UP FAMILY FAVOURITES

Baked beans with garlic

Add a clove of finely crushed garlic and some tomato purée to your baked beans.

Garlic Eggy Bread (Gipsy Toast)

Add some garlic to the egg mix. This gives a subtle flavour to an already delicious and nutritious dish.

Welsh Rarebit

Add garlic to above.

MINCED MEATBALLS WITH GARLIC

125 g (4 oz) minced chicken, turkey, beef or lean pork
oil for frying
2 medium-size garlic cloves, crushed
½ teaspoon grated fresh ginger
½ teaspoon oregano (dry or fresh)
1 medium-size English onion, chopped finely
2 teaspoons tomato purée
plain flour
a small pack of ready-made filo pastry
salt and freshly ground black pepper

Put the meat into a non-stick saucepan with a little of the oil and gently fry until just brown. Add the garlic, grated ginger, oregano and onion. Cook for 5 minutes. Stir in the tomato purée and season to taste. Cook for a further 2–3 minutes and leave to cool.

When cool, turn out on to a floured board and add the flour to thicken and stiffen the mixture. Roll into walnut-size balls and put to one side.

On a floured board, lay out the filo pastry. Cut in squares large enough to take the meatballs. Draw up the corners of the pastry round the meatballs and seal the edges by pinching and twisting, brushing with a little water to seal. Steam the meatballs in a steamer for 30-40 minutes over a pan of boiling water.

Serve with bean sprouts and fried rice with a little soy sauce. If you wish, the meatballs can be served in a little chicken stock.

Serves 2–3

TURKEY BREASTS WITH GARLIC

2-3 garlic cloves, crushed
1 teaspoon each of chopped fresh oregano and basil
1 teaspoon of finely chopped fresh parsley
1 egg white
1 tablespoon cooking sherry (or brandy)
flour
4 turkey breasts
olive oil for frying
salt and freshly ground black pepper

Place the garlic in a glass or china bowl (not metal). Add the oregano, basil and parsley. Add the egg white and sherry. Stir well. Add flour to make a batter-type mix and season to taste.

Place the turkey breasts in the mixture for 1 hour, making sure they are thoroughly coated. Turn regularly. Shallow-fry each side for 5 minutes in the oil until golden brown.

Take out of the pan, put back in the mixture for a second coat and grill for 10 minutes.

Serve with fresh green salad and garlic bread.

Serves 4

HADDOCK AND GARLIC

Ideally you need a large, heavy-bottomed enamel dish in which several pieces of fish can be laid side by side.

4 fresh smoked haddock fillets
milk
6 button mushrooms, wiped
fresh parsley, chopped
fresh oregano, chopped
3 medium-size garlic cloves
2 celery sticks, chopped finely
salt and freshly ground black pepper

Place the fish flat in the dish and cover with milk. Season to taste. Put the remaining ingredients on top of the fish. Place in the oven at 180°C, 350°F, Gas Mark 4.

Remove from the oven and, if you wish add a gratin topping and grill for 5 minutes.

Serves 4

CHINESE COUNTRY CHICKEN

2 tablespoons soy sauce
1 tablespoon sherry
1 tablespoon cornflour
75 g (6 oz) chicken breast, skinned and cut into 1–1.5 cm
  (¹/₂–³/₄ inch) squares
2 pieces of fresh root ginger, about 2.5 × 1 cm (1 × ¹/₂ inch)
  in diameter
4–5 spring onions
2 carrots
4 celery sticks
6 button mushrooms, wiped and sliced thinly
2 medium-size garlic cloves, chopped finely
1 large English onion, sliced
2 teaspoons tomato purée
vegetable oil for frying
freshly ground black pepper

Mix the soy sauce, sherry and cornflour in a small bowl until smooth and creamy. Add a little black pepper to season. Add the chicken breasts to the sauce mixture and stir well until all the pieces of chicken are well coated. Leave to marinate in this mixture, stirring occasionally

Cut the ginger root into matchstick-size pieces and then slice the spring onions into 5 cm (2-inch) lengths, cutting these into thin sticks. Repeat for the carrots and celery. Put the ginger, spring onions, carrots and celery in a bowl with the mushrooms, garlic and onion and add the tomato purée. Put the oil into a small non-stick saucepan and heat gently. Add the chicken pieces to the saucepan and deep-fry until golden brown (about 3–4 minutes). Remove and place on a piece of absorbent kitchen paper to drain. Keep warm.

Take a few tablespoonfuls of the hot oil from the saucepan and put in a wok or a large non-stick frying-pan. Heat until sizzling. Add the pepper, ginger, garlic and onion and stir-fry, keeping the pan as hot as possible. Turn down the heat once all the vegetables have begun to brown. Add the chicken pieces to the pan and cook for a further 3–4 minutes over a gentle heat. Serve with fresh baked bread or hot rolls.

GARLIC SOUP

Cooked garlic, especially when it is boiled, has a subtle flavour that has been described as a combination of boiled potato, chicken and mustard – very gentle and very tasty too. This is a good way to ward off winter ailments – such as coughs, colds and 'flu – or to get rid of an existing cold.

2 whole garlic bulbs
1.2 litres (2 pints) water
a bouquet garni
olive oil
50 g (2 oz) butter
25 g (1 oz) plain flour
50 g (2 oz) parmesan cheese
salt and freshly ground black pepper

Peel off the outer papery membrane from the bulbs and carefully separate the individual cloves. Drop into boiling water and boil well for 30 seconds. Remove from the pan and peel off the outer skins (boiling makes this much easier to do). Place the peeled garlic, water, bouquet garni, a little salt and pepper and the olive oil into a pan and simmer gently for 30 minutes. Then strain the liquid, squeezing the juices from the garlic cloves back into the liquid. Leave to stand.

Melt the butter in a non-stick pan and remove from the heat. Stir in the flour and when smooth add to the soup, stirring while reheating. Simmer for 5 minutes and then serve sprinkled with grated parmesan cheese.

Serves 2–3

5

Garlic for today and tomorrow

Consider the facts. Some 2 billion kg of garlic were grown worldwide during 1988 and 1989 – enough for a medium-size clove for every man, woman and child on earth! Garlic as a cash crop continues to grow in importance and is appearing in the daily menus of millions who until recently would never have thought of eating it. America and western Europe are fast becoming major consumers of garlic, both in diet and as a medicinal material. Alongside this fast-growing acceptance and enjoyment of garlic, come advances in scientific investigation of garlic, which are showing that garlic is indeed a food with many highly beneficial effects on human health. Each of these factors reinforces the other: the more good things we find out about garlic the more we will eat. The more we eat, the more important garlic becomes as a crop and as a medication and the more will be invested in new research to support yet further consumption. Garlic's use is likely to increase astronomically over the next decades, as more people realise that it is a medicine that you can take daily with complete safety. A medicinal food, if you like, that really does work.

GARLIC'S PROTECTIVE ACTION IN DIET

We are all aware of threats to our enviroment and our personal health. Hardly a day goes by without some new enviromental horror story. We are assailed by doubts about the way our food is grown, processed and sold; about the quality of the water we drink and the air we breathe; and a whole host of other actual or potential health hazards we may encounter as we go about our daily business. Simultaneously – almost as though we had discovered it just in time – it appears that garlic has a role to play in protecting us from many of these threats.

The cuisines of warmer countries have always made use of many plants not just to add flavour and colour to their dishes, but also to help to preserve the food and protect against food poisoning. Thus even though 'technological'

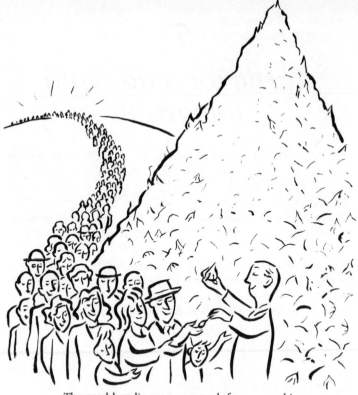

The world garlic crop – enough for one each!

barriers to contamination – such as refrigeration – aren't widely available, use is made of natural ways of protecting from infections. Prime examples of these natural 'antibiotics' are peppers, chilli peppers, root ginger, cloves, mustard, paprika and, of course, garlic.

Many of these plants and herbs are sharp-tasting and highly aromatic and have high oil contents which are known to be both astringent and antiseptic. They are the basis of dishes such as curries, chilli con carne and the countless Chinese recipes which use ginger and garlic. These foods are now widely available in this country and you can add them to virtually every savoury dish you cook, not just for their exciting flavours but also because of their protective benefits.

A large quantity of garlic in your diet can help to kill, or at least render less harmful, any bacterial contaminations in food. Garlic contains potent bactericidal agents, and laboratory tests show clearly that garlic juice, raw garlic, and garlic oils are all able to kill virtually every pathogenic (disease-causing) organism known to science. Moreover, this action is very speedy and completely without side effects. Some of this benefit (which is very pronounced in the raw plant or in its oils) is conferred even after the garlic has been cooked. We know this because the process of extracting essential oils is a form of cooking, using steam to dissolve these precious oils out of the plant material. Yet essential oils have a licence to claim benefit in helping to alleviate coughs and colds – and will undoubtedly help to keep the lungs clear from bacterial infection and to remove any existing infection.

The other area of the body in which dietary garlic can be of real importance is in the digestive tract. Here garlic's antiseptic action is of supreme value in helping to counteract an upset stomach caused by contaminated food or water.

Garlic has also long been used as a preservative for cooked meats in particular and is widely used in China and the Far East as a preservative for summer-picked vegetables which have to be stored for winter use.

So garlic really does give major health benefits when taken in the diet as well as medicinally. Use it every day in at least one dish, and take a healthful supplement too, every day, especially in winter.

It's not only humans who can benefit from garlic's anti-bacterial and anti-viral action, however. Garlic added to chicken feed may help prevent the fowls contracting salmonella[8]: work is now in progress in various university departments to investigate this possibility.

Could garlic be added to the diet of calves to prevent BSE? No one knows at the moment, but it could be another fruitful area for investigation.

We humans, who are higher up the food chain, will directly benefit of course, as we will be in less danger of eating contaminated food.

GARLIC AS AN ANTIBIOTIC
– THE FUTURE

Medical and scientific literature contains a wealth of experimentation on garlic's effects on food-poisoning organisms. This research will undoubtedly be stepped up as a result of our present problems with food contamination. Research will fall into several areas:

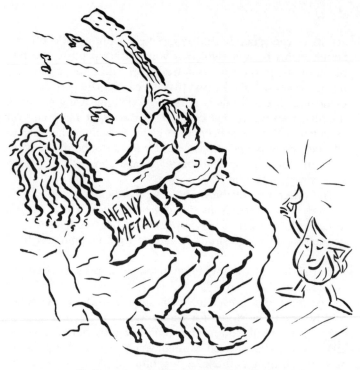

Garlic can combat 'heavy metal' pollution!

- Given that garlic exhibits considerable antibiotic powers in laboratory experiments, what forms of garlic are the most effective?

- What specific parts of garlic's spectrum of organo-sulphur compounds have the highest levels of activity?

- How precisely do these materials act on the bacterium – what are the physical mechanisms that destroy the cell?

- How does garlic neutralise existing bacterial toxins and what are the implications of this unique action?

HEAVY METALS – POLLUTANTS THAT CAN AFFECT US ALL

Garlic appears to be able to reduce the body's concentration of some of the heavy metals, such as cadmium, lead and mercury. Regardless of how careful we are, levels of these substances have been, historically, rising in humans, and they are extremely toxic. Mercury from dental amalgams leaches slowly into body tissues as acids in the mouth slowly dissolve micro-amounts into saliva. Lead contamination is breathed in from car exhausts and can also be ingested in vegetables which have been grown near to roadsides. Cadmium occurs in some concentration in the soils of certain geographical areas and can be taken up into growing plants in high concentrations.

Garlic's ability to claw these unwanted toxic materials out of the system is a consequence of the role of sulphur in stabilising the presence of metallic elements in many body systems. Without the presence in our bodies of sulphur-based compounds arising from our normal diet, many important functions carried out by useful metals in our metabolism simply could not take place. So sulphurs play an important part in the transport and the fixing of beneficial metals in our bodies. It is not too great a leap therefore to view the prospect of the sulphurs in garlic also playing a role in transporting certain toxic or unwanted metals to the organs that can excrete them. In Eastern Europe and Japan, garlic has been used to treat patients who have high levels of industrial metal compounds in blood and tissue with great success. So on this basis alone, in an increasingly contaminated world, garlic should be worth its weight in gold.

FREE RADICAL AGENTS — A POTENTIAL TIME-BOMB

In the process of everyday activity, every cell in our bodies takes in nourishment to produce the energy required to function and make necessary repairs. The byproducts of this energy consumption are water, carbon dioxide and waste products. The constant production of waste-material constantly produces unstable materials called free radicals or oxidising agents, which have to be neutralised by the body. They are responsible for the process of ageing, and for weakening the body's overall resistance to many degenerative diseases. Put more simply, free radicals have an effect on the body similar to what happens when oil goes rancid.

Garlic is believed to mop up these free radical agents and thus render them harmless. It is believed that garlic can actually reduce the production of free radicals at cellular level in the body.

GARLIC AND THE IMMUNE SYSTEM

The human body has a number of strong defences against illness and infection which are collectively known as the immune system. These defences are automatically activated when a threat is perceived. It is believed that garlic helps to excrete heavy metals, which themselves represent a constant and major challenge to the power of our immune system. Constant and repeated threats, such as stress, smoking, poor diet and bad hygiene, multiply the challenges to our bodies' defence systems. The immune system can progressively become less and less effective under the burden of these constant challenges.

But garlic can act as a protective agent for the immune system. We know that garlic has always had a reputation for giving strength and stamina, for warming and drying, for helping to make respiration more efficient and for improving the circulation and oxygenation of our blood. In other words, garlic helps the body's machinery operate with much greater efficiency in many important ways. Such an increase in efficiency takes a heavy load off our immune defences, making us feel healthier and able to resist the next challenge – whether it be 'flu or a tummy bug – much more strongly.

GARLIC AND YOUR CIRCULATION – THE FUTURE

You have read that we have in Britain a dismal record of heart health and are now the 'leading nation' in terms of overall heart and circulatory system diseases. This is undoubtedly due mainly to poor diet, smoking and stress. Do not underestimate the role of stress. The stress of poor environment in terms of bad housing conditions, poverty or stresses in family life can have a direct effect upon your blood! Stress has been shown to make blood platelets more prone to increased stickiness. So worry does have at least one clinically observable effect upon its victims that is of undoubted importance in heart health.

Our problems have not gone unnoticed by the pharmaceutical industry, whose past endeavours to control blood pressure and heart disease have been of great importance to sufferers from these crippling diseases. New drugs are coming which will give even more relief, but they are likely to need to be taken every day and thus to be an ever-increasing financial drain on health resources. Here garlic has the potential to come into its own, as a cheap, preventive medicine.

As you will have seen from chapter 3, garlic's benefits in the maintenance of a healthy heart and arterial systems are well documented and have been the subject of intensive investigation for a very long time. So why has it taken so long for this valuable information to come into the public domain? Cardio-vascular problems are, of course, serious medical matters, and as such tend to be thought of more as the concern of medical specialists than of the general public – unlike more common and less serious ailments such as coughs and colds. This is one reason doctors are often reluctant to share knowledge with their patients – most of whom are untrained in the complexities of physiology and pharmacy – because of the fear that a little knowledge might be more dangerous than none, especially if the information was misunderstood. Neither does the medical profession want to encourage us to do too much in the way of self-diagnosis – in case self-medication is the inevitable result! The danger that a serious hidden health problem could lurk undiscovered behind more minor symptoms for which a layperson is trying to treat him or her self is a serious one. Cardio-vascular disease is one such area of potential danger.

So the first thing to say is that if you suspect that you have any symptoms which could point to problems in this area, you must present them to your doctor. It does appear likely that garlic can offer valuable benefits in the treatment of this family of diseases and that this is becoming increasingly recognised by the medical fraternity. But our purpose is to recommend garlic for its preventive role through diet and self-medication with garlic products. Undoubtedly parts of the wide spectrum of organo-sulphur compounds found in garlic will form the basis of future medicines for use mainly by the specialist in cardio-vascular matters.

Already many heart by-pass patients, people with high blood-clotting potential and people with high blood-fat

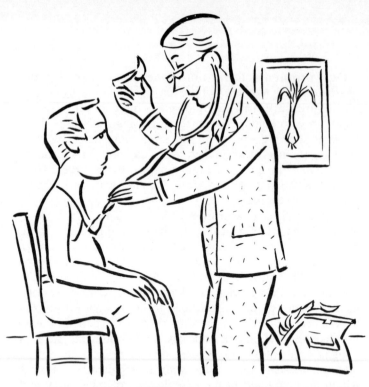

Garlic could be a doctor's best friend!

levels are taking garlic wih the blessing of their practitioners. But the true value of garlic in the curative aspects of cardio-vascular diseases is still, and will remain the province of the dedicated specialist.

Intensive clinical trial work on garlic is now a matter of great importance for many researchers and no doubt will yield yet more supportive results for garlic in the near future.

GARLIC – A SAFE, EFFECTIVE AND NATURAL PLANT MEDICINE

As we have clearly seen, garlic's range of activities is not just confined to the reduction of platelet stickiness, which it can achieve at quite low dose-levels. It also has an effect on the liver and its output of cholesterol – modifying the way in which cholesterol is produced, handled and stored within your body. Garlic is unique in the way that it appears to handle all of the key important aspects of fat metabolism and blood behaviour. No one drug is capable of covering all of these vital areas.

But just as importantly, garlic's safety record is without peer – both as a food and a medication, its record is completely clean. There are no side-effects to be reckoned with, although garlic may be contra-indicated for a few people with low blood pressure or problems with low blood-clotting levels.

If you are sensible enough to follow the advice on how to protect yourself against problems that may arise from bad food, then your bonus will certainly be the benefit of a degree of protection for your heart and arterial system. The same dietary levels of garlic and the same levels of supplementation with commercial garlic products will confer protection.

Platelet stickiness or the tendency of your blood to clot through platelets clumping together will be reduced considerably. But generally, for the beneficial effects on helping your liver to produce more of the HDL fraction which helps to mop up excess cholesterol, you will need just a little more daily garlic to be really sure. Here, I would recommend daily doses of at least twelve tablets taken in three separate doses of four, or three of the one-a-day garlic oil pearles taken separately before the three meals of the day. There is a new oil-filled capsule which contains a high dose of oil (double the one-a-day content, or 4 mg). One of these will help with platelet stickiness but ideally I should take two, one at breakfast time and the other immediately before the evening meal. At these levels you should be able to get a good level of overall protection.

Many of the hundreds of trials on garlic have been undertaken in Third World countries, in which western-style drugs are often too expensive to use widely. Research based on materials which are available locally is much more practical for many countries. Their medical research concentrates in many areas on plant ingredients and the development of dose forms of these for subsequent clinical trials and then for medication. Garlic is a foremost example of this constant search for effective, low-cost, locally sourced medicine. As the world's population continues to grow, and as resources for health care come under increasing pressure, we will be turning to safe, natural, low-cost medicines like garlic more and more, and an important part of the solution to widespread improvements in the level of health around the world might well be here.

GARLIC RESEARCH
– WHERE TO NOW?

Initially garlic must be taken a little more seriously by the healing professions. It is no longer a joke. Medical professionals are already recognising that garlic's benefits are far from illusory, regularly taken and permitted as a daily medication for patients on the ward.

Secondly, although plant extracts are unlikely to be patentable, this should not prevent increasing levels of investigation into garlic's actions. Such work will need to be funded by commercial operations and some initial investigations and projects have already been started, particularly in Germany and Japan. But the main national problem is here in the United Kingdom, and perhaps here is where garlic's potential should be investigated. We live in hope, and as sales of both culinary and commercial garlic rise to new and lofty heights, this will undoubtedly be an important spur to new, high-quality work in our universities and commercial laboratories.

Most of the work showing that garlic is a potent anti-bacterial agent, is done in the laboratory. This doesn't replicate real life, of course, and is only an indicator of activity. We need to know what happens when garlic's useful molecules are absorbed into the bloodstream.

- What is it that's absorbed? Does it change as it travels around the body?

- How many active substances are there in garlic? Are some more effective against one type of organism than another?

- Are the effects of garlic against organisms in the gut the result of garlic materials passing through the area prior to absorption or are they the result of already absorbed active principles within the local blood supply?

There are other important general questions, such as:

- Can allicin be absorbed into the blood?

- As allicin is notoriously unstable above 4°C, how can it ever reach the site of absorption (the intestines) intact?

- Does the application of heat and the passage of time that allicin spends in the digestive system actually cause more robust substances which are true actives for human health to form?

- How precisely can we identify particular fractions of garlic which have specific effects? And so on.

On the cancer treatment front, garlic research, although highly complex, is still in its infancy. But garlic has had a reputation from Egyptian times for use against tumours.

- How real is its potential – does garlic have within it new secrets in the war against this deadly disease?

- Can its regular use at least give some degree of protection?

We don't yet know of course, but there does seem to be a gleam of light at the end of the tunnel.

TAKING GARLIC SERIOUSLY

The foregoing discussion of the state of garlic research shows that the benefits I have been claiming for garlic aren't just speculative ramblings but observations based on research work from all over the world. Garlic is unique in its ability to protect us in so many ways.

So now that you more fully know that garlic is indeed a very serious subject for worldwide research, what can you do to take best advantage of garlic in your daily life?

The answer is very simple. Make sure that you progressively develop the garlic habit. And it is a habit. Once you get used to the flavourful difference that garlic can make to a host of dishes, you will never want to be without it. So get garlic into your kitchen and do it now! When you're feeling a bit below par, have a cold or 'flu or a high temperature, then take a good dose of garlic capsules or tablets. Or make up your own preparations from fresh raw garlic. It can work like magic.

If you have catarrh, a raw clove slowly chewed will banish the problem almost instantly. However, if you're a little wary of the problems of odour and are a gregarious, sociable individual, perhaps pearles or tablets are a better way of taking your medicine.

By now, you shouldn't really need any more reasons to take garlic regularly, but a recap of its benefits might reinforce your determination to get garlic goodness into your life right now.

GARLIC — THE GREAT PROTECTOR

You will have noticed that throughout this book garlic's role has been one of prevention and protection. It can help to prevent you catching a cold because you're run down and susceptible. It can help prevent that awful cough and those aching lungs from turning into something much worse.

Garlic can help to keep your skin clear and healthy and your lungs and stomach in good fettle, whilst preventing mild gastric upsets from many food-contaminating bacteria. Mild mouth infections can be tackled easily with a simple garlic syrup, and there are suggestions that regular dietary garlic helps to reduce the development of plaque-forming bacteria in the mouth (combined with regular teeth-brushing of course!).

But more than this, the known benefits of garlic on your heart and arterial system mean that the sooner you start a garlic regime the better for your heart and your general health. Garlic is the supreme natural medicine – unique in its many modes of action. It's safe, inexpensive and easily available. If modern pharmaceutical scientists discovered a new ingredient that was only a tenth as capable as garlic, they would be delighted!

I hope you will agree that the future of garlic looks almost as exciting as its remarkable past. Garlic is now, after thousands of years, making a home for itself here in the west. Soon everyone will take garlic for granted – as much a part of daily diet as the potato! But what we should never take for granted is garlic's ability to help improve our health and protect us against disease.

Appendix A
A window on current garlic research

Admittedly only a small window, but the following areas of investigation into garlic's abilities are taken very seriously these days. Whilst you are already aware of the vast arsenal of research work that is already being undertaken into garlic's role in cardio-vascular disease and gastro-intestinal infections, the following summaries of published papers take us into some of the other none-the-less important areas of human health in which a role for garlic is already perceived as more than a mere possibility. Some of this work is at the forefront of its field, and you will be forgiven if some of it is a little difficult to follow, but I shall do my best to explain what the investigator was up to!

Over the past three years, some 200 or more investigations into garlic's actions, its chemistry and its potential for yielding important new compounds have been published in leading medical and scientific journals. Today, the pace is if anything accelerating and in 1989 alone, over 60 papers were accepted for publication by the world's medical and agricultural academic press.

Mutation Research, 1989; 227: 215–219 Zhang et al. of Zheijang Medical University, Hangzhou, China. 'Antimutagenic Effect of Garlic on 4NQO Induced Mutagenesis in *Escherischia coli* WP2'.

Escherischia coli is a bacterium found universally in the human gut. It can be responsible for infections of the urinary tract and so on. It is very commonly used in research of this nature. Mutagenesis is a change in a gene which could incline the carrying cell to become cancerous. In this trial two agents, ultraviolet light and a chemical agent, were used to induce a gene change. Extracts of garlic were shown to prevent the gene changes in the bacteria exposed to chemical assault. They were, however, ineffective against the changes caused by ultraviolet light. This paper is basic research, but even at this stage perhaps a valuable pointer to the direction in which research could be going.

Planta Medica 1989; 55: 506–508 Horie T, et al. Tokyo College of Pharmacy, Japan. 'Protection of Liver Microsomal Membranes from Lipid Peroxidation by Garlic Extract'.

Microsomes are ultra-microscopic components of cells and possess lipid or fat-based membranes. The possibility that so-called free radicals might be involved in their peroxidation (damage by oxygen) is exciting a great deal of interest at the moment. Free radical injury has been tied in with many diseases and is certainly a component of the ageing process.

In this trial, extracts of garlic were able to prevent some of the chemical and physical changes that occurred when rat livers were deliberately challenged by lipid peroxidation. This area is one of enormous complexity, and proving anything that might directly relate to human organs is exceedingly difficult. This piece of research gives another pointer to a direction in which research into garlic extracts will undoubtedly be going in future.

Journal of Biochemical Toxicology 1989; 4: 151–10 Belman et al. Institute of Environmental Medicine, New York, USA co-authored with Eric Block and George Barany. 'Inhibition of Soybean Lipoxygenase and Mouse Skin Tumour Promotion by Onion and Garlic Components'.

This study found that certain components of garlic's essential oils inhibited chemically induced and promoted cancers of mouse skin. Induction is the first stage in a cancer's development, and promotion is the second stage, in which a cancerous state has actually occurred. This paper also reviews in some detail much of the work that has clearly demonstrated inhibition of the development of skin cancers (which were deliberately promoted using chemical carcinogens) through several specific components found in onion – but more particularly in garlic. Again this excellent paper clearly indicates the path along which garlic research in this area of human disease will proceed.

Anti-Cancer Research, 1989; 9: 273–27 Jang, J J et al. Cancer Centre Hospital, Seoul, South Korea. 'Effects of Allyl Sulphide, Germanium and NaCl on the Development of Glutathione S-Transferase P-Positive Rat Hepatic Foci Initiated by Diethylnitrosamine.'

Again this paper concerns the use of carcinogen

(Diethylnitrosamine) to initiate pre-cancerous changes in rat livers. Here again, garlic showed the ability to modify beneficially the progress of these changes and a possible mechanism for the way in which garlic extracts might work is given. Components of garlic appear to inhibit selectively a cellular material (cytochrome P-450) which is a key motivating candidate for the activation of the primary cancerous changes in the liver cells under investigation.

Asia Pacific Journal of Pharmacology, 1989; 4: 133–140 Sumiyoshi, H & Wargovich, M J. Garlic (*Allium sativum*): A Review of its Relationship to Cancer.
The essence of this wide-ranging review of much of the published work to date is summed up as follows:

> 'The precise inhibitory mechanism of garlic on carcinogenesis (the commencement of the cancer-forming cellular changes) has not yet been characterised .....constituents of garlic are slowly being revealed to be excellent experimental inhibitors of both the initiating and promoting phases of carcinogenesis.'

Here again cytochrome P-450 is mentioned as being inhibited by garlic and identified as a key component of the process by which cancer begins.

Oncology, 1989; 46: 277-280 Nishino, H et al. Kyoto Prefectural University of Medicine, Japan. Anti-Tumour Promoting Activity of Garlic Extracts.
This paper shows that garlic extracts can inhibit the first stages of tumour promotion in two-stage mouse skin carcinogenesis. This promotion is achieved using a chemical (TPA) which acts by increasing phospholipid metabolism at an early stage of promotion – but garlic extracts actively inhibited this increased metabolism. Again this paper points us in a similar direction to the majority of recent research papers on experimental inhibition of cancer formation with garlic compounds.

Cancer Research, 1988; 46: 277–280 Wargovich, M J et al. Department of Medical Oncology, University of Texas, USA. 'Chemoprevention of N-Nitrosomethylbenzylamine-induced

Oesophageal Cancer in Rats by the Naturally Occurring Thioether Diallyl Sulfide'.

This is a potentially important piece of work in which the authors have used a chemical carcinogen (NMBA) to induce cancer of the gullet in rats.

Animals which also received Diallyl Sulfide at the same time as attempted promotion of carcinogenesis, however, showed no signs of microscopical cancerous lesions nor any spreading changes. The garlic extract was also shown substantially to reduce the hepatic (liver) microsomal metabolism of NMBA. (This material has to pass through the liver where it is converted using the cytochrome P-450 already mentioned in two previous papers.) The authors comment that it remains to be seen whether directly acting carcinogens such as nitrosamines would be inhibited. In other words does the garlic component also have a protective effect on the gastro-intestinal tract walls? The paper by You, which follows shortly, proposes that there may indeed be the prospect of such a protective effect from regular consumption of garlic.

Environmental and Molecular Mutagenesis, 1989; 13: 357–365 Knasmulle, S et al. Institute of Experimental Cancer Research, Innsbruck, Austria. 'Studies on the Antimutagenic Activities of Garlic Extract.'

This paper presents further evidence that garlic possesses anti-mutagenic properties (and by extension anti-carcinogenic capabilities).

It shows that extracts of garlic reduced the lethal effects of gamma irradiation on *E. coli* (mentioned in a previous summary) and on strains of *Salmonella typhimurium*. Another extract of garlic inhibited fat peroxidation induced by hydrogen peroxide – again in bacterial subjects.

Journal of the National Cancer Institute, 1989; 81: 162–164 You, W C et al. Beijing Institute for Cancer Research, Peoples Republic of China. 'Allium Vegetables and Reduced Risk of Stomach Cancer.'

This is a widely quoted paper, a study of the reality of people's lives in terms of dietary habits and their consequences. This study observed an area of China where gastric cancer rates were high. The researchers interviewed 564 patients with stomach cancer and a further 1131 people who had no cancer, as a control. They were able to show that there was a significant reduction of the incidence of stomach cancers with increasing consumption of allium vegetables (mainly garlic and onions). Those in the highest quarter of allium consumption ran only 40 per cent of the risk of those in the lowest consuming quarter. It appears to have been a very well conducted and monitored trial.

Next we move on to new work on garlic's role in helping to control fungal and bacterial infection.

Journal of Applied Bacteriology, 1990; 68: 163–169 Hannoum, M A, Faculty of Science, Kuwait University. Inhibition of *Candida* adhesion to buccal epithelial cells by an aqueous extract of garlic.
This paper shows that exposure of the *Candida albicans* species (responsible for thrush) to an aqueous garlic extract reduces the adherence of the bacteria to the lining of the mouth. This adherence is the initial stage in the development of candidal infection. Besides incubating the extract with the fungus to demonstrate the effect, the author also studied the consequences of rinsing the mouth with differing concentrations of garlic extracts. These tests too showed a significant reduction in adherence to the mouth linings. The author notes that live yogurt mixed with fresh crushed garlic does appear to give relief to sufferers from oral thrush. This paper shows that garlic may be a valuable first line of defence against this condition.

Chem Pharm. Bull. 1988; 36: 3659–3663 Matsuura, H et al. Wakunaga Pharm Laboratories, Hiroshima, Japan. A Furostanol Glycoside from Garlic Bulbs of Allium sativum l.
The authors have isolated a new glycoside from garlic and shown that it inhibits the growth of *Candida albicans*. Its activity however, was much less effective than the anti-fungal drug generally used to treat this condition. The author notes that the safety and tolerance which attaches to the use of garlic can ensure that high doses can be given without harm whereas with fungicidal drugs great care has to be taken to ensure that no adverse reactions occur.

Now on to some recent work on garlic as a cardio-vascular medicine.

Journal of Food Safety, 1989; 9: 201–204 Subramonium, A, et al. Central Food Technologies Research Institute, Mysore, India. Influence of Certain Dietary Plant Constituents on Platelet Aggregation.
In this paper, dietary constituents were used in human blood samples deliberately to induce platelet aggregation.

This was reversed with the addition of garlic juice. As we know, compounds which counter aggregation have a protective role against thromboembolic disorders.

Appendix B
Useful addresses and references

Mersley Farms, Newchurch, Isle of Wight, PO36 0NR
Write to the above address for supplies of top-quality seed corms, giving your name, address and postcode, with the quantity you want to order. At the time of publication, prices were as follows:
1 dozen: £2.50
2 dozen: £4.00
3 dozen: £5.50

United States Tourist Office
22 Sackville Street
London W1X 2EA

The Garlic Research Bureau
PO Box 40
Bury St Edmunds
Suffolk IP31 2SS

1. Buck, Donner and Simpson 'Garlic oil and ischaemic heart disease' *International Journal of Epidemiology* II, 1982.
2. Ariga T, Oshiba S, Tamada T 'Platelet aggregation inhibitor in garlic' *Lancet* 1:150, 1981.
3. Chutani SK, Bordia A 'The effect of raw versus fried garlic on fibrinolytic activity in man' *Atherosclerosis* 38:417, 1981.
4. Sharma KK et al 'Effect of raw and boiled garlic on blood cholesterol in butterfat lipaemia' *Indian Journal of Nutritional Dietetics* (1976) 13, 7.
5. Boullin DJ 'Garlic as a platelet inhibitor' *Lancet* 1:770, 1981.
6. Zheziang Institute of Traditional Chinese Medicine 'The effect of essential oil of garlic on hyper lipemia and platelet aggregation' *Journal of Traditional Chinese Medicine* 6:117, 1986.
7. Symposium of the chemistry, pharmacology and medical applications of garlic, 23–25 February 1989, Lüneberg, West Germany *Cardiology in Practice.*
8. Johnson and Vaughn 'Death of *Salmonella typhimurium* and *E. coli* in the presence of freshly reconstituted dehydrated garlic and onion' *Applied Microbiology* 17, no. 6, 1969.

Index

abscesses 15
  tooth 11, 60, 63
acne 66
ailments curable by garlic 32
allicin 35–6, 37–8, 44–5, 59, 60,
  86–7
Allium sativum 7, 51
animals and garlic 10, 17, 46, 56–8
antibiotics, drug-based 19, 29, 46,
  47, 48, 62, 63
'antibiotics', natural 78
  garlic as 'antibiotic' 78, 79–80
antiseptic qualities 46
arteries
  ageing 60
  blockage 23
  congested 23
  'furring-up' 22, 27
  'hardened' 22, 23
  narrowing 26, 94
  walls of 22, 27
atherosclerosis 22, 27
athlete's foot 66, 67

bacteria 16, 29, 69, 88
  beneficial 29, 47, 63, 69
bacterial infection 15, 16, 46–8, 79
bactericide, garlic as 15, 16, 46–8,
  78, 80, 93
bites and stings, 66, 67
blood, 'thinning' of 14
blood-clotting 38, 41, 44, 83–4, 85
  low level of 85
blood-fat levels 34, 35, 40, 43–4, 58,
  83–4
blood platelets 22–3
  aggregation 42, 43, 44, 94
  clotting 22, 23, 37, 42
  stickiness 27, 28, 33, 34, 35, 38, 42,
    82, 84, 85
blood pressure 83, 85
breath odour 31, 64, 66, 70, 88
bronchitis 13, 30, 50
Buck, Donner and Simpson study
  24

cancer 21, 50, 62, 87, 90–3
candida 47, 93
catarrh 13, 21, 30, 50, 64, 88
children and garlic 61–2, 65, 66
cholera 10, 16, 47
cholesterol 25–7, 40–1, 84, 85
clinical trials *see* garlic research
cold sores 67–8
colds 10, 21, 49, 50, 60, 65, 76, 79,
  87, 88
corns 48

coughs 10, 21, 49, 60, 64, 76, 79, 88
cramp 14
cysts 67

deodorised products 61
Di Allyl Disulphide 37, 42
diarrhoea 60, 64–5
diet 22, 23, 24, 82
digestion 30
  of garlic 36
digestive organs/tract 64, 79
doctors/GPs 58, 63, 65, 83–4, 86
dysentery 19, 47

essential oils of garlic 37, 42, 43–4,
  45–6, 60, 66, 79
excretion of garlic 30
  by mucous membranes 30
  through the lungs 30, 31, 47
  through the skin 30, 57

fats
  mono-unsaturated 25
  polyunsaturated 25, 28
  saturated 24, 25, 27, 28, 35, 40, 41,
    70
  unsaturated 25
fats, animal 22, 28, 66
Festivals of garlic 55
fibrinolitic activity 38–40, 44
food contamination 69, 78, 79, 88
food poisoning 69–70, 77
free radicals 81–2, 90
fungicide, garlic as 53–4, 93

gangrene 13, 19
garden, garlic in the 53–4
garlic, cooked 5, 37, 70
  boiled 40–1
  fried 38–9
  taste of 76
garlic, raw 36, 38–41, 42, 50
  suggested daily intake 45, 59
garlic extract trials 42–6
  oil 42–4, 45–6
  powdered 44–5
garlic growing 51–3
garlic products 5, 58–61
  daily doses recommended 59, 85
  deodorised 61
  essential oil, 60, 79
  oil-filled capsule, high dose 85
  one-a-day doses 61
  pearles 60–1, 85, 88
  powders 59
  tablets 59, 85, 88
  when to take 70

garlic research
clinical trials 33–5, 62, 84, 85
reports of 38–41, 42–3, 89–94
future questions 79–80, 86–7
gastric upset 60
in children, caused by garlic 62
gastro-intestinal tract 29, 69, 89, 92
German requirements 59
growing garlic 51–3
gut infections 46, 48, 69, 96
in animals 46

heart disease 10, 22–7, 44, 62, 82, 83, 89
High Density Lipoproteins (HDLs) 27, 44

immune system 49, 50, 81, 82
infants and garlic 62, 65
influenza 21, 49, 65, 76, 87
insects and garlic 11, 19, 30, 53–4, 66

jaundice 17

leprosy 10, 16
liver, human 25, 27, 84, 85
longevity 9–10
Low Density Lipoproteins (LDLs) 27
lungs 30, 31, 49, 79, 88

malaria 11
Methyl Allyl Trisulphide (MATS) 37, 42, 43, 46
mouth infections/ulcers 65, 88

oil of garlic see essential oils
onions 24, 41, 90, 93

pets and garlic 56–8
platelets see blood platelets
Ploughman's Lunch 41
pneumonia 13
pollutants 80–1

preservative, garlic as 77–8, 79
Product Licence 21, 49, 79

raw garlic see garlic, raw
recipes with garlic 71–6
remedies, garlic 63–70
research see garlic research
respiratory tract 14, 16, 46, 48, 63–4
rheumatism 10

salmonella 56, 63, 79, 92
scientific methods/research 13, 20, 33, 77, 86–7; see also garlic research
sinus/sinusitis 30, 49
skin 50
clearness of 88
elimination through 30, 57
garlic applied to 65–6
infections of 16, 31, 46, 48, 66
rash, caused by garlic 66
smoking 22, 23, 28, 82
sore mouth 47
sore throat 47, 63–4
stamina 14, 16, 82
stomach upsets 62–3, 64–5, 79, 88
stress 22, 23, 28, 82
strokes 23
sulphur compounds 30–1, 36, 37, 46, 48, 51, 60, 61, 70, 80, 81, 83

thrush, oral 93
tonic, garlic as 65
tooth abscesses 11, 60, 63
tuberculosis 10, 47
tumours 10, 87, 91
typhoid 10, 47
typhus 16, 19

verrucae 48, 68
virus infections 48–50

warts 48
worming agent, garlic as 10, 17, 57